Bless This House

Creating Sacred Space
Where You Live, Work & Travel

Mama Donna Henes

ixia
PRESS

Mineola, New York

Bibliographical Note

Bless This House: Creating Sacred Space Where You Live, Work & Travel
is a new work, first published by Ixia Press in 2018.

Library of Congress Cataloging-in-Publication Data

Names: Henes, Mama Donna, author.
Title: Bless this house : creating sacred space where you live, work &
  travel / Mama Donna Henes.
Description: Mineola, New York : Ixia Press, 2018. | Includes
  bibliographical references and index.
Identifiers: LCCN 2018001669| ISBN 9780486818450 (alk. paper) |
  ISBN 0486818454 (alk. paper)
Subjects: LCSH: Sacred space. | Space—Religious aspects.
Classification: LCC BL580 .H46 2018 | DDC 203/.8—dc23 LC record
available at https://lccn.loc.gov/2018001669

IXIA PRESS
An imprint of Dover Publications, Inc.

Manufactured in the United States by LSC Communications
81845401   2018
www.doverpublications.com/ixiapress

*For Omar, who will always live
at home in my heart.*

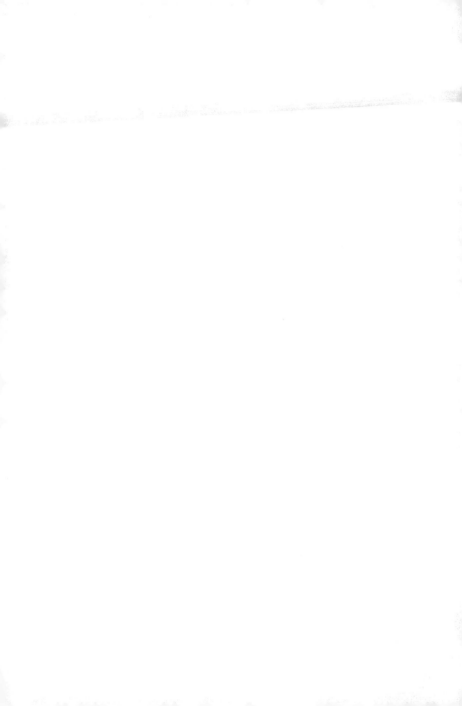

A home is a symbol of the world, our own mini-world, our own Mother Earth. When we feel safe and comfortable in our homes then we feel more able to deal with the outside world. When we remember this link consciously and honor our homes, we will change our relationship, not only with our homes but also with our wider home, the planet herself.

—Jane Alexander, *Spirit of the Home*

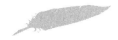

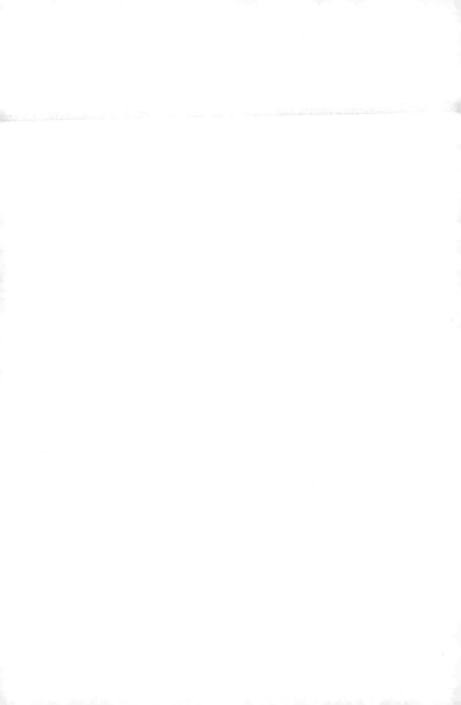

CONTENTS

ACKNOWLEDGMENTS

My heartfelt appreciation and deepest gratitude to Deirdre Mullane, my agent and dear friend, who has always seen the worth of my work and stood by me through exciting thick and depressing thin. To Nora Rawn, my incredibly smart, perceptive, compassionate, and generous editor, and to the entire tireless team at Dover for providing me with a most supportive, pleasant, and satisfying publishing experience. To Sarah Reynolds, my amazing multitalented assistant who always knows everything I don't. To Jimmy, Tommy, Terry, Terry, Andre, Dennis, Ed, Ryan, Paul, Marsha, and Sarah, my old building mates cum family, who taught me about the true meaning of home: about belonging, mutual acceptance, support, and unconditional love. And always, always and forever to Daile for absolutely everything important.

INTRODUCTION

Stay, stay at home, my heart, and rest;
Home-keeping hearts are happiest.
—Henry Wadsworth Longfellow

House Mama

My home houses Mama Donna's Tea Garden & Healing
Haven, my ritual practice, which includes blessing
ceremonies for weddings, funerals, new babies, new
homes, and new businesses. Of all the ritual services I
perform, my most popular requests are for space clearings
and aura uplifting. I have cleansed and blessed the energy
in hundreds of domiciles of every description and social
stratum, in commercial and corporate environments, and
for film, television, and Broadway productions. I have also
worked with realtors to create an inviting atmosphere
in the places that they are showing, and to stimulate
movement in previously unsalable properties.

It is my intention in writing this book to share my
love, knowledge, and long experience of creating and

maintaining a sacred energy in any space, so that anyone anywhere can be inspired to cleanse and bless the atmosphere in your own homes and work spaces. *Bless This House* gives you the nuts-and-bolts wherewithal to establish the environment you want, and to do this creatively and effectively.

Here is a comprehensive suggestion manual for DIY (do-it-yourself) house blessers. It offers extensive practical information about tools, supplies, and procedures to use, and it covers all the Whys, Whats, Whos, Whens, Wheres, and Hows of the clearing and blessing process. There are detailed lists of cleansing and blessing agents: descriptions, prescriptions, benefits, and explanations of how and when to use them. There are, as well, fascinating and inspiring examples of multicultural House Blessing traditions, as well as prayers and blessing words from many spiritual paths to help you express your own personal domestic needs and desires in a ceremony that you create to bless your house.

Bless This House is also in part a spiritual guide to individual empowerment. It offers a series of personal examples and stories, inspirational texts, poems, quotations, folklore, and questions to contemplate, designed to stimulate your reflective process and heighten your awareness of your space and how you relate to it. This will help you to identify how your home feels to you and how you want it to feel and to function. This introspection leads to trust in your instincts and inner knowings and your willingness to act on them.

Above all, *Bless This House* urges you to claim psychic ownership of the energy that surrounds you. It fosters your confidence that you have the authority and the ability to establish a living environment for yourself and your family that is safe, supportive, and comforting and feels great. The resulting blessing ceremonies that you create will reflect your feelings and intentions, your personal taste and style, and your philosophy and belief traditions. Your personal House Blessings will ensure a uniquely resonant energetic atmosphere that is deeply meaningful, incredibly powerful, and always, always perfect.

Blessings to you and your home.

xx Donna Henes

A true home is one of the most sacred of places.
It is a resting-place to which at close of day the
weary retire to gather new strength for the battle
and toils of tomorrow. It is the place where love
learns its lessons, where life is schooled into
discipline and strength, where character is molded.

—J. R. Miller, *Home-Making*

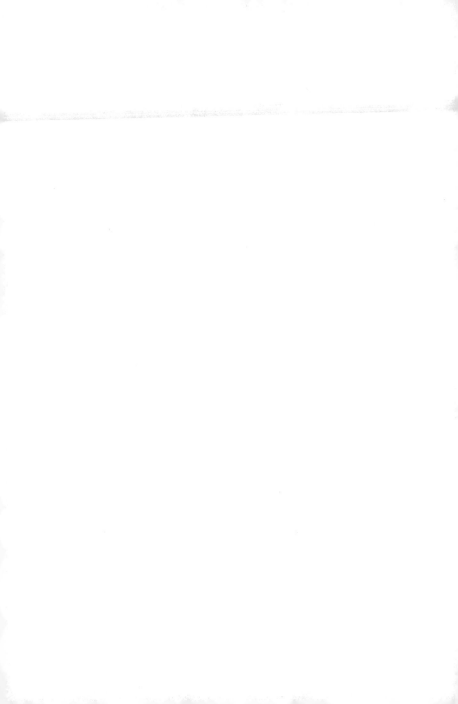

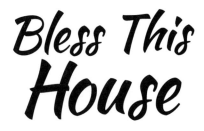

Bless This House

CHAPTER 1

There's No Place Like Home

I am a homebody. I have been a devoted dyed-in-the-wool homebody since my very first home of my own, an extremely raw and slightly scary storefront loft in a tenement building on the Lower East Side of Manhattan. I loved that place and especially loved that it was a large empty space just waiting for my creative expression. I was an art teacher, after all. What fun! I took great pride and pleasure in taming some of the most deplorable aspects of this ugly barn and creating an environment that was quirky and funky and mine, all mine. This was my exciting grand adventure Maiden Loft. I would probably never have left this living project-in-process, had it not been for the fire in that decrepit building that left me homeless.

That first exuberant experience of loft living was followed by a two-year period of having to live in furnished rooms, because I had lost everything I owned in the fire, and of course at twenty-two years of age I had no insurance. Then I lucked out by being able to sublet a loft in the Garment District from an artist who was in England for a couple of years. I could not make any permanent changes to her living environment, but her huge workspace was empty and available for temporary transformation. Having this much space to create in was my dream come true and led to my early forays into the art world. Alas, the owner returned home one day unannounced, six months early, and again I had to move on a dime.

The only place I could find on such short notice was a five-thousand-square-foot loft with no heat and no hot water in an old factory building in downtown Brooklyn. There were two remaining factories in the building and the other five floors were empty. The building owner was so nonplussed that I wanted to move in and actually live there, he gave me the first three months' rent for free. Imagine: fifty feet by one hundred feet totally empty, with fourteen windows on three sides. Since I still owned nothing, I moved into this abyss with a hibachi for cooking and heat and a foam mattress for furniture. Period.

The first few years were a true hands-on hard-hat experience, but eventually the space was made livable. Little by little, with a lot of help from my friends, I created an environment that was fluid and flexible, serving as playground, studio, office, laboratory, disco, classroom, meditation room, bathtub room, ritual space, and performance space, as needed. This loft, and the eclectic community of creatives who eventually moved in and became family, stimulated my artistic growth and spiritual transformation. Here I raised cats, dogs, and birds; art, spirit, and consciousness; and a dear young boy. This was my Mothering Loft, where I lived for seventeen fabulous fruitful fun years, and I probably would be there still, had the building not been taken over by a developer who evicted all of us by rule of eminent domain.

The next, and hopefully the last, move brought me to a loft under the eaves in an old Victorian school building deeper into Brooklyn, near Prospect Park. I have been here for nearly thirty years now and pray to never have to leave it. This is my mature Queen Loft, the expression of all I have learned about having, losing, leaving, and staying home. I know who I am and what I like and want and need to surround me. I have it, because I have created it. And I created it, because I needed it. This House of Many Altars is the self-portrait of my soul. Here is my heart. Here is my spirit. Here is my home. Here is my life. It offers me everything I need to be centered and productive, serene and happy. It suits me, inspires me, soothes me, and pleasures me with beauty, sanctity, reverence, and gratitude. And because it holds three decades of blessings, the aura that it exudes is powerfully palpable to everyone who enters. It just feels really good here. That's the goal, isn't it?

> Home is the nicest word there is.
> —Laura Ingalls Wilder, *Little House on the Prairie*

In the beloved children's novel *The Wonderful Wizard of Oz*, when the homesick farm girl Dorothy Gale closes her eyes and chants, "There's no place like home. There's no place like home," she's not thinking about the actual structure that she grew up in, its architectural form, decorative details, or how many rooms it has. She's recalling the haven of safety and cheer that it provided for her. Her nostalgia is fueled by happy memories of Auntie

Em's home-grown, home-cooked meals and home-made quilts, Uncle Henry's protective husbandry, the toasty house-bound winter nights they shared, and all the other cozy comforts that made her feel loved and secure. That modest Kansas abode, along with the family, farmhands, and animals that lived there, is home to her soul.

The idea of home is as old as humanity itself. Our most ancient ancestors were mostly nomadic, finding or creating shelter as they roamed in search of food. Like burrowing animals, they took cover in caves and under overhangs, and like nest-building birds they made lean-tos and dugouts for protection from the elements. These temporary domiciles offered a certain amount of physical safety and comfort, but primarily they provided a focus for communal connection. Even a small campfire in the vast dark wilderness can feel like home when it reflects the faces of the people you love.

While today we often think of a home as a physical place, a specific edifice and geographic location, it remains, more than anything else, an emotional refuge. Homer's epic eighth-century BCE poem, *The Odyssey*, chronicles the decade-long journey of Odysseus as he makes his way home from the Trojan War. The weary, homesick soldier opines, "There is nothing more admirable than when two people who see eye to eye keep house as man and wife, confounding their enemies and delighting their friends." Pliny the Elder, a first-century Roman naturalist, philosopher, and naval commander, also suffered long, sad separations from the comforts, community, and conviviality of home. He penned the famous proverb "Home is where the heart is."

Eighteen hundred years later, Lord Byron echoed that thought when he wrote, "Without hearts, a home is not a home." The English word "home," itself, reflects the connection between heart and home. Home is derived from the Middle English word *hām*, which means "village, hamlet, manor, estate, dwelling, house, region, country." "Home" referred mainly to a gathering of people, and only secondarily to the actual place where people gather. An early definition of the word "house" referred to "family, ancestors, and descendants." Home *is* where your heart is, surrounded by the hearts of those you know and love and trust. As Oliver Wendell Holmes put it, "Where we love is home—home that our feet may leave, but not our hearts."

The term "home" still elicits a profound archetypal emotion that expresses the universal human need to belong. Home is an expansive concept, bigger, broader than the boundaries of our personal domiciles. Home includes the people, buildings, and nature that surround us—our neighborhood, our community, city, state, and country. Home extends ever outward in a complex matrix of concentric circles rooted in mutual recognition of connection, identification, and allegiance. In urban parlance, fellows who share the same familiar turf, experiences, and ethos refer to each other as "homeboys," "homies," or "homes." They are members of the same home team that offer comradely understanding and support.

> To dwell means to belong to a given place.
> —Christian Norberg-Schulz, *The Concept of Dwelling*

In Japan, the members of Yakuza societies are also bonded by their connection and allegiance to the same home area. The literal meaning of *yakuza* is "rooted in a territory, taking care of that territory." The Yakuza refer to themselves as *ninkyō dantai*, meaning "chivalrous organizations," with a centuries-old ethic of looking after their local communities. Despite the violence they wield in the course of their mafialike crime business, they are valiant in their sense of responsibility for the welfare of the home front. They were the first responders in both the 1995 Kobe earthquake and the tsunami of 2011, arriving with supplies and aid well before the government emergency services were mobilized.

That feeling of belonging also holds true for those who live alone. In the United States, where there are more than 33 million single households, 28 percent of the population lives alone, but they inhabit homes nonetheless. In Sweden, where 47 percent of people live singly, a study of "The Multiple Meanings of Home as Experienced by Very Old Swedish People," published in the *Journal of Environmental Psychology*, found that for people eighty to eighty-nine years old and living alone, home represents both security and freedom. To have one's own home is to retain one's independence. As someone who loves living alone, this rings very true to me even though I am not yet in my eighties!

Home means security because it is where we feel we belong. It is familiar, functional, and filled with layers of memories and personal belongings that both reflect and define us. It is ours as we have made it. Home is our protective place where we can prepare to go out into society, and the safe, private place where we can return to our own personal world for repose, reflection, restoration, and personal expression. Home feels safe, because we make the rules and the decisions that affect us. We can decide whether and when we want privacy, solitude, and quiet or if we would welcome the company of others, and if so, who and for how long.

There is safety in that autonomy, and great freedom, as well, to really live as we choose. In our changing society, where so many people live alone, our home does not house our family; rather, it *becomes* our family, generating intimate, almost personified welcome, acceptance, refuge, warmth, and emotional support. The poet Patti Smith lives a very private solo life. In her memoir, *L Train*, she writes, "Home is a desk. The amalgam of a dream. Home is the cats, my books, my work never done."

When people are asked to define home, they do not generally speak in terms of architectural style, building materials, comfortable amenities, or even location. They talk about how they feel there. Home refers to a place that is safe, that offers nurturance, hospitality, and communion, and that supports self-confidence, self-development, and personal expression. This applies to all ages, even young people, who we often think of as living in the private virtual reality of their own personal electronic devices. In an article published on theodysseyonline .com, college students listed their feelings about returning home for a visit during a break in the school year, and they all focused on home as a secure source of nurturing, cushy comfort, and organized order after having lived in disorderly, uncomfortable, and unpalatable dormitories:

- "Good-bye cafeteria. At home you have a full-size refrigerator filled with more than just beverages and frozen dinners, a pantry housing your favorite snacks, and a complete kitchen that doesn't smell like the one in the dorm's basement."

- "The bed is softer, the couches softer, the carpet is softer, the towels are softer, even the toiletries are softer! After living the conventional-over-comfort style of dorm life, home feels like a pillow palace."

- "No alarm to set. The only other thing that can wake a college kid up in the morning is the smell of food made specially for me by Chef Parent."

- "Those few days and nights go by in the blink of an eye. While you're excited to go back to see your friends, it's bittersweet to leave your loved ones and the comforts of home. You just have to get through the horrors of Finals Week and you'll be back before you know it. Dorothy had it right though, 'There's no place like home'."

Many of these young millennials come out of college with no job and an enormous student debt, making it impossible to establish a home for themselves as a newly minted adult. The American dream of finishing school, moving out of the family home, and getting a house or apartment of your own is now indefinitely deferred. This situation has created a mass migration of kids returning to their parents' home to live once again with their families while they work and save enough money to finally fledge the nest. This is a practical solution, to be sure; however, it is a significant intrusion on the life plan of the parents as well as the child, rife with potential problems and irritations for both.

The child is no longer a child and chafes at having parental rules again after experiencing the relative freedom of a student. The parents have gotten used to having an empty nest and find that they like it just fine now that it is their turn to attend to their own needs and desires. Perhaps the old childhood bedroom has been converted to a space for their own enjoyment, which could make the returning progeny feel unwelcome in what had always been their home. And if the childhood bedroom is still intact, living there can be infantilizing for the kid, and create a care-giving burden for a parent who had been enjoying more freedom than in decades. Although a certain mutual resentment, expressed or repressed, is understandable, it has the potential to create discomfort for all concerned. But then again, some families adapt admirably to the current reality by being flexible and adjusting their habits and attitudes to accommodate each other in a new way that assures that everyone's needs are being met. In this way, they are reclaiming the family home as a place of safe haven, welcome, and mutual respect.

> Perhaps home is not a place but simply
> an irrevocable condition.
> —James Baldwin, *Giovanni's Room*

The wonderful Spanish word *querencia* captures this metaphysical concept. The *querencia* is the safe place in the bullring where a wounded bull will retreat to gather his strength and gear up for a fresh charge. *Querencia* is defined as "a place where one feels safe, a place from which one's strength of character is drawn, a place where one feels at home." In his touching piece for the *New York Times*, "Where is Cuba Going?," the writer John Jeremiah Sullivan defines *querencia* as "an untranslatable Spanish word that means something like 'the place where you are your most authentic self'." Home is where you know who you are.

Querencia, home, provides a supportive atmosphere that is at once soothing and energizing, enriching, inspiring, and healing. It is the embracing nest that comforts and nurtures the well-being of our body, mind, and spirit, where we can develop and grow. It is a chrysalis-like spiritual shelter, a cozy cocoon in which to think and dream, plan, create, and evolve. Where we can truly inhabit our best selves. And it is the durable shell, the protective refuge where we can retreat, recharge and rejuvenate, repair our psyche and restore our balance. Our *querencia* is the welcoming port in the storm, offering shelter, warmth, and comfort. The fiercer the storm, the more comforting it is to be home. Ideally, our home is like the carapace of a snail or a turtle that we carry on our back and in our soul wherever we go. When we feel nourished, peaceful, and safe at home, it is so much easier to feel the same way when we are out in the world.

Whatever else home is, it is the starting point of how we define ourselves. It is the center of our world and the axis mundi of our reality. Home is where our most personal lives happen and where we are most authentically our truest self. Home is home base, home plate, homeroom, hometown, homeland, homestead, "home, home on the range." Without a home, we are not only without shelter, we are without connection, rootless. No longer grounded, we are like poor little lost E.T. riding his bike through space, pitifully keening "Home. Home. Home," unfettered, uncentered, unhitched and unhinged, lost in a turbulent cloud of unreality with no light signal to guide us to port.

DREAM HOUSE

Because they constitute such a large part of our waking lives, dreams of houses are a common theme for the unconscious mind. House dreams are nearly universal, experienced regardless of gender, culture, geography, religious or spiritual beliefs, and time and place. According to Carl Jung's system of dream analysis, the home is a primal symbol for the Self, composed of your mental, emotional, physical, and spiritual parts, just like your house is divided into rooms that each serve a different purpose. Quite an apt metaphor. Your body houses your soul, after all. "Home is like a house inside your head where your thoughts gather," writes Marcus Eriksen in *My River Home*, his memoir of returning from war.

Dreams of home offer rich insights to help us discover and integrate hidden and underused parts of our Self. A Chernobyl refugee evacuated from the region explained, "During the day we lived in the new place, and at night we lived at home—in our dreams."

My own dreams of home are always a grand adventure that involves exploring strange houses of every description or looking through my own home with new eyes. My nocturnal treasure hunts reveal hidden attics, secret doors, mysterious passageways, treasure chests with hundreds of drawers, each one housing jumbles of phantasmagoria, wondrous items and images, incongruous juxtapositions very much like the artist Joseph Cornell's marvelous boxes. I am always discovering some hidden gem, some new idea or insight, a sudden revelation, a new appreciation, or sometimes, when I am really lucky, a completely composed poem, essay, or chant. Obviously these dream houses symbolize the maze brain of a shaman, a writer, an artist, a healer, a seeker, a seer. They help me to explore the labyrinthine recesses of my soul in search of wisdom and enlightenment. "Our soul is an abode," wrote Gaston Bachelard in *The Poetics of Space*, "and by remembering 'houses' and 'rooms,' we learn to 'abide' within ourselves."

There are the houses we visit in our sleeping minds, and those we daydream of, castles (or studios or cabins) in the sky. These might be practical in nature, imagining different ways of arranging furniture in your own rooms or those of a new house, or they might be wholly invented fantasies, spaces to house your different identities or your ambitions. If your own dream house represents your psychic state, what does it look like?

- Is your house built with a single story or many floors?

- Is there an attic? A basement? A garden?

- Is it spacious or cramped?

- Is it dark and gloomy or sunny and bright?

- Is it an open floor plan or are there separate spaces?

- Are the rooms empty or full?

- Is it cluttered and messy or neat and organized?

- Is it filled with all your favorite things?

- Is it sturdy or shoddily built?

- Does it make you feel house-proud?

- Is it well taken care of or showing neglect?

- Is everything in it in working order?

- Is it in need of home improvement?

And, more important, what do you *want* it to look like?

- Try drawing or writing or singing or dancing the image of your dream house.

- Picture it.

- Picture it with you there.

- Picture your dream house as your self-portrait.

- Feel its aura.

The more you think about these questions, the more able you will be to take emotional and spiritual ownership of your home and create a feel-good energy to nourish, comfort, and inspire you, your family, and anyone who enters there. As you read, keep in mind this dream vision of your ideal home to guide you.

Home was not the place where you were born but the place you created yourself, where you did not need to explain, where you finally became what you were.
—Dermot Bolger, *The Journey Home*

Your home is yours. You are welcome here.

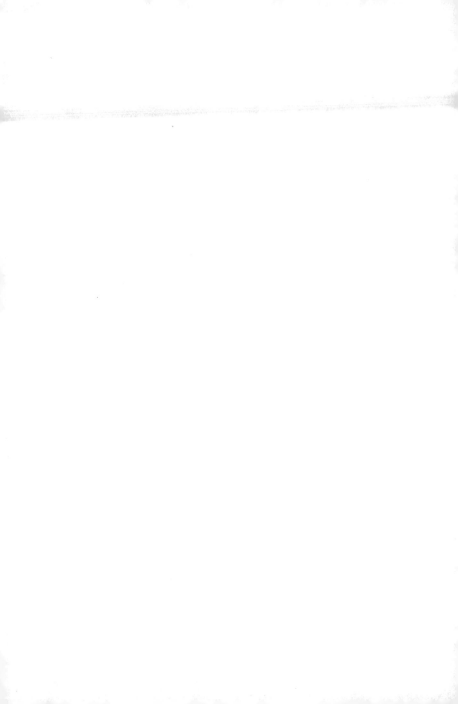

We shape our dwellings, and afterwards
our dwellings shape us.

—Winston Churchill
Sir Winston Churchill: A Self-Portrait

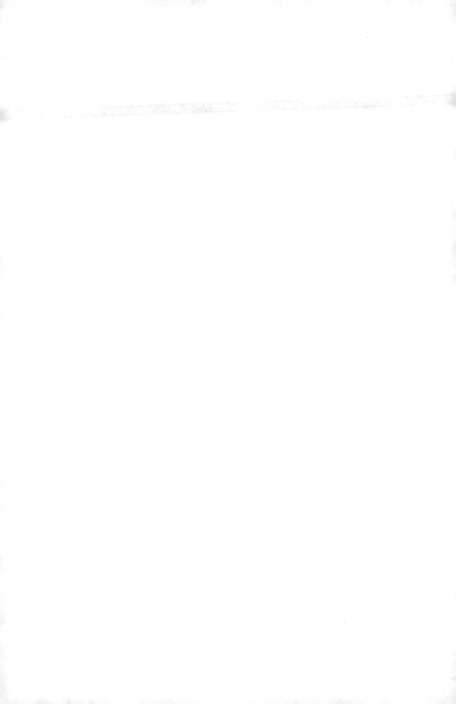

CHAPTER 2

Homing In

Your dwelling is the psychic as well as the physical space that you occupy in the world. It houses your body, your energy, your thoughts, your moods, your demeanor, your spirit, your deeds, and your legacy. Your home is your most intimate space—so it is vitally important for you to feel good there. You want to be in harmony with your surroundings, comfortable, secure, relaxed, at ease, at home. Your house should be your solace, your safe place, your *querencia*—your nest, your burrow, your hive, your cave, your den, your cocoon, your carapace. It is your go-to port in the storm that shelters you and those you love.

Your dwelling gives you a firm foundation beneath your feet, and it keeps your head dry when it rains. It fulfills your physical needs, providing you with warmth, with space, with security. Shouldn't the energetic atmosphere within its walls support you emotionally and spiritually as well? Your home is your castle, your refuge, your sanctuary. And if it isn't, it should be.

But what if it's not?

WHEN IT'S TIME FOR A HOUSE BLESSING

Occasionally, for any number of reasons, the environment in your own house might not feel especially hospitable to you. Everyone has worries and stress, problems of every description. Everyone experiences change, planned or arbitrary, welcomed or not so much. All of this irritation, disappointment, upset, or resentment encountered in the course of your day is sure to spill over and dampen the atmosphere in your home, which both reflects and affects the people living in it. Our hardest times of life have an even more traumatic effect on our environment. Dark or disruptive energy in your closest quarters is extremely depleting—mentally, physically, emotionally, and spiritually. Tempers flare, depression sets in, and accidents can happen when the environment is unbalanced. The good vibes that you want in your most intimate space become heavy and thick, which in turn limits your best spirits. Simply put, bad moods create bad energy in the home and bad energy in the home creates bad moods. It can be a reinforcing cycle.

> People and the places where they reside are engaged in a continuing set of exchanges; they have determinate, mutual effects upon each other because they are part of a single, interactive system.
> —William S. Sax, *Mountain Goddess*

If for any reason the energy that surrounds you feels negative or blocked, sad, scary, or stale, it will have a damaging impact on the atmosphere in your home. Consequently, when you find yourself in the deepest throes of anxiety, depression, fear, sorrow, suffering, or loss, when you most need warm and calming domestic support, your home may not have the right energy to lift and sustain you. Living in a space that does not feel right ultimately affects your state of mind, your health, your relationships, your productivity, even your finances. Troublesome energy in your home is contagious and will infect everyone who encounters it.

But you can remedy that toxic situation. It is, after all, ultimately up to each one of us to create the environment in which we want to live. You can clear and cleanse your environment spiritually as well as physically like you do with mop and broom. A house cleansing and blessing ceremony will accomplish the task whether you are just settling into a new place or refreshing the home that you have been living in.

MOVING IN

House Cleansing Blessings performed upon taking a new residence are as old as houses themselves. They have been, and still are, practiced in every spiritual and religious tradition in the world. It is widely customary to perform ceremonies to clear the space of unwanted energy before moving into a new home. Blessings for new domiciles vary in their details from culture to culture, but all House Blessings are intended to sanctify the home and shower its inhabitants with love, luck, health, abundance, and protection from harmful energy. Blessings cleanse any negativity and infuse an abode with uplifting, life-affirming positive spirit that will support and sustain those who live and visit there. A critical time to cleanse and bless your residence is right when you are ready to move in.

Moving, even in the best of situations, is always unsettling. Leaving old friends, familiar places, landscapes, and activities is not easy. Sometimes a move is required in order to deal with an upsetting shift in circumstances, such as the loss of a job, a divorce, a death, a natural disaster, any of which creates additional levels of anxiety. According to some surveys, moving is third, after the death of a spouse and divorce, on the anxiety meter. No matter the cause, moving always involves a huge amount of work to prepare, pack, and transport your life, lock, stock, and barrel, and then settle into new digs. Major stress! Moving to new living quarters is one of life's most emotionally loaded and disruptive experiences for most people, because it brings up a deep-seated dread of being uprooted and not belonging.

But moving can also be among the most exciting, hopeful, and rewarding of life experiences. In India, moving into a new home carries ritualized importance that is second only to weddings. Moving represents a new beginning, a fresh start, a new lease on life. A new home is the headquarters of the next chapter in your life, so you will want to consecrate it with all the hope, expectation, and optimism that you feel by performing a spiritual cleansing in addition to whatever housecleaning you will do. This clearing removes the residual energy left by all of the previous residents, builders, contractors, inspectors, and potential buyers or renters and replaces it with your own. Blessing your new abode invites in all goodness that will nourish your life. This is a great way to stake a claim to your space, to plant your desires and intentions for living there, and to create a psychic boundary to protect its sanctity. Blessing your space will transform a new house, apartment, or room into a home. *Your* home.

Habitat for Humanity and other service organizations that build and renovate houses for those in need finalize the completion of each project with a dedication ceremony, during which all the volunteer workers gather to bless the new house and officially turn over the keys to the relocating family. The blessing is meant to honor the work and giving spirit of the many folks who made the new home possible by sharing appreciation and thanks. In this way an attitude of gratitude charges the energy in the space and inspires the new residents to build on their own sweat equity by reaching out to help others. The volunteers are also empowered by the process. Fonda Rush, the executive director of the Lauderdale County Habitat for Humanity, says, "When you see the families work so hard to get into a new home and what a new home means to them, stability of their family, stability of their life, it is just really rewarding. And you also know that you've accomplished something that God has asked us to do and that's to care for our neighbor." The circle of giving and receiving *is* the blessing.

Here is the opening and closing prayer from a beautiful Dedication Key ceremony for a new Habitat for Humanity house built entirely by women:

Opening Prayer

As we draw together this evening, let us pause for a moment to remember the faces of the many women who have gathered in this space to build a house for <name>. Let us remember the women who have shared of their spirit, their energy, their wisdom, and their time to help another realize her dream of not just receiving a house but creating a home. In bringing together the spirit of love, the gift of service, and a renewed hope for one family, these women have consecrated this ground and made it holy.

Today, we bless more than a structure. We bless <name> as they move into this house built by the dreams and labor of generous, wonderful, and wise women. It is <name> who will complete the project. Only they can bring that final ingredient which will make this house a home. Their love as a family will reverberate through these walls for years to come. It will become a fixture that will hold them in their joy and celebration as well as in their sorrow and tears.

And so in the spirit of life and love ... we bless all those who gather.

In the name of all that we, in our separate traditions, deem holy and sustaining, we bless the many gifts of Women Build, this home, and the <name> family.

...So may it be, amen.

Closing Prayer

May the love that lifted the rafters
And hung the shingles
ripple out into the community of Chatham
and return on the waves along the shores of
    Cape Cod.
May the love that grew in fellowship of a
    common goal
continue to grow in the lives of <name>

…as they grow together in laughter and tears,
joy and sorrow.
And when the day is long and life is hard
may they feel that same love as they pass
through this door.
may they know that they are held in care by a
much larger community
may they know they are guided by something
much greater than themselves.
And, may those that gather today and in the
days past, know that their love has indeed
blessed the life of another.
This is indeed the house that love built.
May that love keep shining.

You can adapt this to make your own dedication ceremony for a new home.

MOVING ON

It is also a good idea to clear and recharge the energy of a place in your preparations to rent or sell it. If you yourself are moving on from your current residence, it's smart to remove accumulated energy generated by your family and friends in order to neutralize your personal domain and direct a clear energy flow that will make it seem more appealing to future residents.

Realtors are seeing the benefit of revitalizing the atmosphere in the houses and apartments they are showing. Staging has become a popular practice in advance of having an open house to show a property. This is done to create an anonymous environment, a blank canvas so that potential buyers can visualize their own lives in that same space. In addition to clearing away personal items and creating a neutral color palette and spare visual aesthetic, it is crucial to also remove any residual troubled or stuck energy that lingers and "colors" the atmosphere.

A Space Cleansing and House Blessing before putting a home on the market will clear the air and allow for new ownership in a place that *feels* (and not just looks) welcoming and comfortable. The newly energized and cleansed atmosphere attracts buyers on a very visceral level. I have seen this work again and again. Invariably, previously unsalable houses and apartments—even those that have been on the market for months and years— will sell soon after performing a cleansing and blessing ceremony in them.

"Thank you so much for helping me with the house last night. Cameras and TV stuff aside, I feel much better about being in the space now that you've been through it. You have a calming presence that the house needed."

—Ryan Serhant, star of *Million Dollar Listing New York*

THINGS CHANGE

The driving need to balance unsettling energy is deeply felt and sometimes feels so urgent that it can seem like an emergency. A few years ago, I got a call from a harried television producer, who told me in confidential tones that one of the stars of her very popular program believed that her home was cursed with negative energy. She was afraid to stay in the house any longer, but was also reluctant to move. She was desperate. Could I do anything to help? the producer wondered. "Sure," I replied. "That's what I do."

Imagine my surprise upon learning that the show she was referring to was "Mob Wives," the popular Reality TV show. Since I had never seen this program before, I watched a few past episodes online. Based on the back-story, dense with deception, despair, disgust, and divorce, I knew that the energy in her house must be truly awful.

So, I headed out to Staten Island to help Mob Wife Renee Graziano clear away all the demon energy that was draining her life force.

After assessing the situation at the house, I delved deeply into my blessing bag arsenal. I used sage and cedar, to smudge away the brutal betrayal and pent-up rage. I burned sweetgrass liberally so the sweet smoke would refresh the dampened spirit of the place and invite in all the sweet spirits. I burned some tobacco as an offering of gratitude for the good gifts the house has brought her and her son. Then I blessed Renee and her home with fragrant oils and sprayed all the surfaces with water mixed from fifty holy healing wells from around the world. In the end, Renee, who was nervous, cautious, and perhaps a bit resistant at first, experienced a huge healing, a palpable spiritual realignment caught on camera. It really was Reality TV! Afterward, she told a reporter, *"I just needed to cleanse my house of all the bad things that were going on at the time, so I called Mama Donna to clear the space. It almost felt like a complete turnaround. The air felt thinner. It didn't feel so miserable. After it was done I could laugh again."*

The spiritual environment of a home is created communally by the people who live there; consequently, any shift in the circumstances of any one person can disturb the delicate balance of personalities and perspectives that contribute to the general feeling of a place. And any change in the living arrangements in the home can, in turn, create a stressful atmosphere for everyone in the household. Even a wonderful development—a new relationship, a new roommate, a new baby, a new pet—can shake up the status quo, agitate the energy, and throw you off kilter. Schedules change, needs change, moods change.

Whether you are newly partnered, newly parented, newly single, blending your family with a partner's, or encountering an empty nest, accommodations to your accommodations need to be addressed—energetically as well as physically. It is a good idea to clear away any tense or resistant energy to these shifting circumstances and bless the transition. A House Blessing will consecrate your shifting circumstances and create an optimistic and flexible attitude that will support these adjustments.

Life changes sometimes require that either the house itself or some of its rooms be altered, renovated, or redecorated in order to fulfill a new function. The new baby needs a nursery, so you make alterations to the TV room. You have moved to a new location and want to be able to host visiting family and friends, or you invite your in-laws or grown children to move in with you and they need a private space, so you finish the basement and fit it out with a kitchen and bath. Your new spouse has three children, doubling the kid population in your house, so the attic will have to be transformed into a dormitory and playroom. Your company allows you to work from home, or you start a business of your own and you and your staff need an office, a studio, a consultation room, or a workshop, so you park the car outside and fix up the garage. In every case, a blessing will create a warm and welcoming atmosphere for the new inhabitants and an energetic boost to the new activities that will take place there.

If your nest empties out, leaving you with room to spare, you can now convert a child's old room into a sanctuary for yourself—a room of your own in which to pursue your own passions, whether practicing your violin, painting, weaving, scrapbooking, sewing, exercising, meditating, studying, napping, daydreaming, or writing the great American novel. But in order for this room to provide the creative and productive environment that you crave for your own pleasure and pursuits, the parental energy that you previously projected when your kids slept there needs to be recharged with your own personal renewed desires and intentions. After the dust has cleared, the fresh paint has dried, and the furniture has been installed, a blessing can bring good luck and positive energy into the repurposed space.

THINGS HAPPEN

In addition to the endless list of potentially positive changes in living arrangements, life has a way of also handing us difficult situations to deal with in our homes. Shit happens. Sometimes life changes over which you have no control can infect your home with fear, friction, conflict, and strife. Financial conditions may worsen, leaving you beset with anxiety and stress. The state of affairs at work, in your relationships, or in the world at large might affect your good humor and leave you with crippling worry, anger, or depression.

Roommates and family members may project their own distress onto each other and argue in an unending back-and-forth blame game. Kids can act out their sibling rivalry by constantly bickering in a maddening manner. Couples might fight about unresolved resentments or everything and nothing at all, and eventually separate. Any of these situations will certainly create a most unpleasant toxic environment. Despite the popularity of all the television shows about haunted houses, the most common disruptive energy in a home is not paranormal at all, but created by the very real emotions and state of affairs experienced by the people who live there. And as time goes on, each change of circumstances in the house calls out to be blessed in order to help those affected to adjust and adapt. Blessings help us make the best of whatever life presents or become more proactive in changing what does not work for us.

At one time or another we are all faced with hard times, bitter circumstances, trouble, and tragedy. Hard life changes and painful situations brought about by illness, depression, discord, divorce, and death all have a devastating effect on the atmosphere in your home or place of business. Sometimes the circumstances are so excruciating that they decimate any feelings of comfort and safety that we might otherwise cling to. You or someone in your household could (heaven forbid) fall ill, in which case your house will need to function as a nurturing sick room, a cheerful convalescent home, or a serene hospice. A spiritual blessing of the space can help enormously to enhance the healing process or facilitate the peaceful passing of a loved one by providing an atmosphere that is calm, comfortable, and energetically supportive, both to the patient and to those who serve as caregivers.

It is crucial to remove the heavy, oppressive weight of fear, suffering, and loss that weighs on us in challenging times. The process of cleansing and blessing your environment will help you to process your deeply upset emotions and to rebalance the energy that has been so painfully disrupted. Once the challenging energy has been released, you can bless your house with a renewed spirit that can help foster emotional healing, understanding, and peace of mind. Such a ritual creates a safe milieu where closure and regeneration can take place, providing an atmosphere of hope and the possibility of positive new beginnings.

> If the doors of perception were cleansed everything
> would appear as it is, infinite.
> —William Blake

At their best, blessings increase our fortitude against adversity and loss. I recently received an email from a woman whose husband is in the final stages of his disease. He is receiving hospice care at home and he will die there. She asked if I could come on the day of his death to bless his soul and hers before the funeral home comes to take his body away. She wanted a private, intimate ceremony of farewell while he was still in the bed, in the room, in the home that they had shared for so long. She was also planning a more traditional memorial service that would include their extended circle of family, friends, and colleagues a few weeks after his cremation. In addition, she requested that, once the memorial was over and his ashes were scattered according to his wishes, I perform a thorough House Cleansing and Blessing ritual. Her intention is not to erase his energy, nor her cherished memories, but to clear the space of the heaviness of his suffering and her sorrow, and to consecrate the house for the next stage of her life on her own.

Space clearing and blessing is called for any time that shifting domestic circumstances cause deeply felt emotional reactions, feelings of uncertainty or unease, confusion, conflict, or upset. A blessing ceremony will remove any unwanted, uncomfortable, or blocked energy; purify the atmosphere that surrounds you; and invite in a lighter, energizing spirit, which will make you feel comfortable and safe. A House Blessing will also revitalize energy that is stagnant and stale and remove any psychic blocks to manifesting home as haven. Protecting your home and your emotional state by clearing the energy will reduce your stress level and boost your sense of security and satisfaction. Once your space is cleansed, it will no longer seem unsettling. Your house will become the welcoming safe space that you deserve.

RITUALS

Times of gathering, celebration, and pleasure also deserve to be sanctified. Blessing your space before any social occasion—receiving dinner guests, hosting a family get-together, or throwing a party—creates a warm, cordial environment that conveys your desire to be hospitable. Hospitality is defined as "friendly and generous behavior toward visitors and guests, intended to make them feel welcome," and it is linked etymologically to host, hostel, hotel, hospice, hospital. Hospitality is a highly regarded value in virtually every culture. The general idea is to offer courtesy, comfort, sustenance, and protection to those who are far from home—as the Swahili proverb admonishes, "Celebrate with your visitor as much as you would like to be celebrated."

> Hospitality is a form of worship.
> —*The Talmud*

Comfort is a vital aspect of what makes home feel like home. Comfort implies welcome. Years ago a new friend invited me to her apartment for the first time. It was an extremely uncomfortable visit, both physically and emotionally. There was no room for me in her home. Literally. Not that her space was so small, but because she lived like a hermit and had one chair, one cup, and one glass. It was not because she had just moved in and had not yet unpacked. She had been living there for some time. And it was not because she was poor. She was gainfully employed. She was perfectly polite. She offered me the chair and sat on the windowsill. But when it came to creating and sharing a welcoming and comfortable energy—for herself or anyone else—she was clueless. We continued to see each other, but mostly at my much more convivial house. Happily, today, decades later, she is a fabulously gracious and generous host. We must consciously choose to make our homes hospitable.

After hosting a gathering, once the guests have gone and the house has been put back into order, you might want to cleanse your home of any residual energy that has been left behind by your company. This is not to say that your home is polluted by the scary, harmful energy of your visitors. But we all have our stuff, our worries, concerns, ailments, and complaints. You have enough of your own. You don't want to take on any aggravation, anxiety, or upset from anyone else.

Not even from those you love dearly. Open the windows, burn fragrant herbs, clear it all out and refresh the energy of your environment so that it is now once again charged to serve your personal, private life.

There is nothing like staying at home for real comfort.
—Jane Austen, *Emma*

Since debilitating, enervating energies have a way of accumulating over time, it is a good practice to perform periodic clearings to refresh your space on a regular basis. Clutter, hoarding, and messy habits block energy flow, which results in a claustrophobic, stale atmosphere of agitation, indecision, and confusion that can stop you cold and prevent you from living a full and satisfying life. Make it a habit to clear away anything in your space—physical, mental, emotional, or spiritual—that does not serve you or that stands in the way of your growth and fulfillment.

In fact, all it takes to make your customary house-cleaning regimen into a spiritual clearing is your intention to make it so. House Blessings are wonderful for imbuing your surroundings with your desires and intentions. It is a way of rededicating the space and your relationship to it.

While you mop the floor, be mindful of removing tainted energy as well. Along with an application of wax, you can add a liberal amount of positive spirit to keep helpful energy flowing in your direction and support you as you walk through your day. You can renovate and restore the spirit that surrounds you in the same way you might apply a fresh coat of paint.

Time to dust again
Time to caress my house
To stroke all its surfaces
I want to think of it as a kind of lovemaking
...the chance to appreciate by touch
what I live with and cherish.
—Gunilla Norris, *Being Home*

The *New York Post* has referred to me as an "A-List Exorcist," but space clearings are not always about eradicating hostile, painful, or frightening energies. They are also important when our living and working spaces feel dense, stuck, or stale, especially after a closed-in, stuffy winter, which I suppose was the Old Wife's reason for establishing an annual Spring Cleaning regime. When our grandmothers tackled spring cleaning, they scrubbed everything, *every* thing, inside and out with a vengeance. Their goal was to erase dirt and dust, for sure, but also to release any thick, sticky, unsettling energy that had gathered over the winter. Since windows were not opened for several months, they knew that the atmosphere inside was stale, stuffy, and stifling. Enervating. The dead air was capable of sapping the strength of the family. So they opened all the windows to let the accumulated stagnant energy escape and also to invite in the revivifying vernal spirits of birth and life and growth.

At the start of each season, and at the New Year, gather your clan and, individually and collectively, perform a seasonal House Blessing to release whatever you do not wish to carry into the next period with you. Clear away everything on every level—mental, emotional, physical, and spiritual—that does not further your sense of well-being, personal growth, and loving family dynamics. Remove the mess and dirt and consciously lighten any accumulated disappointments, clinging resentments, bad attitudes, failures, and destructive behavior. Abolish the old, the worn out, the stuck and sluggish energy. Let it all go. Make room for the new. Now you can bless your home and everyone who lives and visits there with the refreshed energy of the new season, the New Year, the new cycle, the new start. Take advantage of these special opportunities to create and dedicate a spirited home environment that can nurture you and serve your needs now and as the future unfolds.

As you near the New Year, it is only natural that your thoughts turn to new beginnings, new possibilities, and new hope. Now is a good time to evaluate your past experiences, actions, and reactions to prepare yourself mentally, physically, and spiritually for your future. Your reflections and resolutions for change at this transition period from one year to the next are critical, for they create the ambient atmosphere and attitude that will surround you and support your personal spirit and the spirit in your home environment for the entire year to come.

A new year, a new season, a new day represents another chance, a fresh start, a clean slate. All over the world, houses are scrubbed spick-and-span from top to bottom and yards and walkways are swept spotlessly clean in preparation for the New Year. In Hong Kong, ten days before the New Year, women observe a Day for Sweeping Floors. At this time, an intensive house cleaning is begun in readiness for the New Year. Nothing, no corner, is left untouched. In Myanmar, the former Burma, the New Year festival of Thingyan drenches the entire country, every building and dwelling and all of its inhabitants, in cleansing water. In old England, New Year's Day was the annual sweeping of all chimneys. The expression "to make a clean sweep" comes from this New Year's custom.

Cleaning house to make ready for a new year is a universal task, symbolic and reverent as it is practical. Out with the old and in with the new! Death to dirt! Removing the dust and detritus accumulated during the previous year ensures the ridding of a dwelling and its occupants of the shortcomings and disappointments delivered during that time, as well. Domestic renovation signifies spiritual and social renewal.

A House Blessing is always appropriate any time when things "just don't feel right." The home is a psychological metaphor for the Self. Blessings enhance the ambience in your home. They simply make the place feel good and you feel good in the place. Your body dwells in your house and your body houses your spirit. "Your house is your larger body," as Kahlil Gibran wrote. So if your home does not feel right, you cannot feel right. The Dalai Lama says, "Cleansing your environment is a ritual means of also cleansing your mind." When you cleanse your environment and put your house in order, you are, by extension, purifying your soul.

I know this sounds rather daunting, but help is at hand. The following chapters offer lots of information and inspiration to help you visualize, create, and conduct a personalized, meaningful blessing ceremony for your home. Keep reading!

May your troubles be less
Your blessings be more.
And nothing but happiness
Come through your door.
—Dorien Kelly, *The Last Bride in Ballymuir*

*This is your home.
It absolutely needs to feel right!*

We all have within ourselves a blueprint
for just the home that will shelter our spirit.

—Victoria Moran, *Shelter for the Spirit*

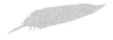

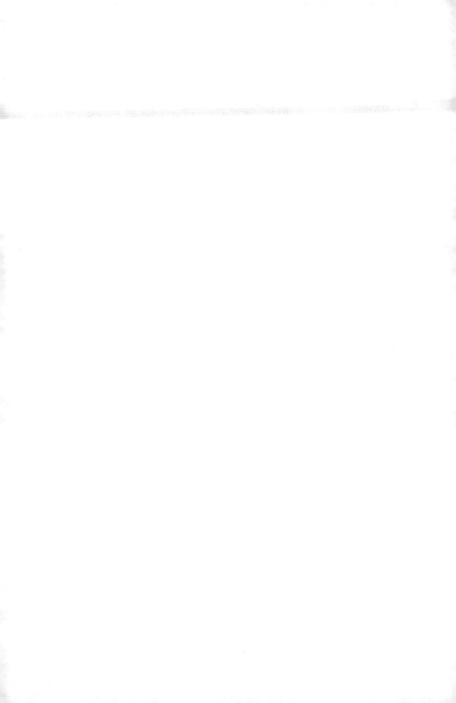

CHAPTER 3

Home Making

When you settle into a different house, apartment, or room, the new space becomes the setting for a new chapter in your life and the incubator in which you will grow new memories. So it is worthwhile to contemplate what this move represents to you, and what you want to accomplish while living there. In her book *Feng Shui for the Soul*, Denise Linn writes, "Your home can be much more than a mere shelter and a repository for your belongings. It can be a magical place where dreams are conceived and realized, where relationships grow and blossom and where problems are tackled and resolved. Ideally your dwelling is a place you want to come home to, where you invite guests, express yourself and feel nurtured by those you love."

It is ultimately up to you to create an atmosphere that expresses your vision of the perfect home for you. What are your hopes for your new home? How do you envision its purpose? How do you plan to use it? How can it serve your needs—body, mind, heart, and soul? What are your intentions for your space?

- A stable residence to protect and nurture your new or growing family?

- A downsized dwelling for a more manageable life?

- A welcoming home base to return to after traveling?

- A party place to host convivial celebrations and gatherings?

- A pleasure palace in which you can indulge your senses?

- An inspiring environment to encourage creative pursuits?

- An organized space for productive work and/or concentrated study?

- A fixer-upper project to challenge your skills and give you purpose?

- A womb room for protection, safety, and security?

- A comfortable and comforting refuge for nurturing and healing?

- A serene sanctuary for quiet meditation and private retreat?

Take some time to think about the ambience that you want to create in your new home. Draw on elements you enjoy from the homes of friends and family, as well as from your own past homes.

- Does the overall atmosphere there make you feel welcome and comfortable?

- Does the space itself, as well as the furnishings and objects that fill it, reflect your vision and intention of how you want it to be?

- Can you feel the rightness or wrongness of the energy that surrounds you? When you can feel this in your bones, do you use that information to identify what to accentuate, and what to avoid?

Once you reflect on these questions, you will know in your heart and in your gut what changes would make your place feel the way you want it to feel. You know how you feel and what you need. You know what you want. You know what feeds you and what defeats you.

You know what you know; you just need to listen to that inner wisdom.

We are what we think.
And that which we are arises with our thoughts.
With our thoughts, we make our world.
—Buddha

The best way to create the very environment that you envision in your new dwelling is to consecrate the space and bless it to house your new beginnings. In this way you can eradicate any stagnant energy, the leftover atmospheric footprint of previous occupants, and replace it with your own optimistic desires and positive intentions. Out with the old and in with the new! By blessing your space, you claim it and make it your own.

The first spirit cleansing and blessing that you perform in your new abode will set the energetic stage for the life that you will live there. Bless your home to make it whatever and however you want it to be. Bless your vision of domestic support for your most deeply felt needs. Your blessing will create a harmonious and nurturing environment that will shelter, sustain, and support you and yours, as well as those who come to visit. Your blessings will make your new house your home.

Nourish beginnings, let us nourish beginnings.
Not all things are blest, but the seeds of all things are
blest. The blessing is in the seed.
—Muriel Rukeyser, *Elegy in Joy*

Your new home will probably not stay quite as pristine and shiny as when you first moved in, and your original blessing will not last forever, either. Eventually after time passes and you and your home experience the normal ups and downs and accumulated detritus of daily life, you may sense some shift, some subtle discomfort or discord in the feeling of your home. The environment where you eat and sleep, rest and work, play and dream may no longer radiate the easy comfort and joy that your initial blessing generated. The steady balance of your home space, and your heart space, has been disturbed. You might find yourself feeling ill at ease and craving the once-sweet spirit that seems to have soured. Now another cleansing and blessing for your much loved, much lived-in home is called for.

"How can I be sure if the energy in my home isn't right?" you may ask.

It's simple: Intuition.

You do not need to be psychic to tell if the energy in your home is light, airy, cheerful, serene, and secure, or not. How does it feel? Trust me, you will know! Or better yet, don't trust *me*. Trust yourself. Trust your feelings and instincts, your own inner knowing. Trust your gut. Our gastric system, our twenty-foot-long labyrinthine gut, uses thirty neurotransmitters, as does our cerebral brain, and it contains some one hundred million neurons, more than in either the spinal cord or the peripheral nervous system, earning it the moniker of Second Brain. This second brain assesses our true felt-in-the-pit-of-our-stomach gut-level emotions and sends these visceral sensations to the brain in our head, which then tells us in so many words what feels right and what does not feel right.

It is easy to recognize when your home needs physical repair or renovation, or when your decor and furnishings need to be refreshed and revived, because you can actually see the wear and tear with your own eyes. You certainly know when it is finally time to tackle the accumulated clutter in your rooms when it begins to present a danger of injury if you trip. You know when it is time to tidy up when you keep misplacing things in the mess. Be confident that it is equally clear and obvious when the energy that surrounds you needs to be revitalized. Energy is like air. You can't see it, but you can feel it. Learn to pay attention to your psychic surroundings just as you notice peeling paint or lurking dust bunnies. If it doesn't feel right, then it isn't right. It is as simple as that.

This is your home. It is speaking to you! Listen to it. Take a tour around your space and pay attention to what it is telling you as you pass from room to room. What does it want; what do you want? What does it need; what do you need? Are your original intentions for new beginnings still evident? Or has your house moved away from you? Does your home still satisfy your needs?

Your home is your partner in life, and contributes to the life you build there. In fact, you cocreate the ambience of your abode *with* your abode. Listen to your home and listen to your own inner voice. How does it feel to you? How does the energy that you feel in your home affect you? How do you contribute to creating the energy that you feel? How would you like to feel when you are at home? How do you want others to feel when they are there? What energy does your place need to have in order for it to feel right to you? Does it feel

- Safe?

- Comforting?

- Comfortable?

- Depressing?

- Stimulating?

- Calming?

- Dark?

- Light?

- Bright?

- Orderly?

- Chaotic?

- Cluttered?

- Expansive?

- Cheerful?

- Claustrophobic?

- Welcoming?

This process of self-examination will enable you to identify your intentions for your space and to claim the confidence and authority to enact them and accept the responsibility (or response-ability) for manifesting them. Trust your feelings and instincts about what energetic changes are needed in your most intimate environment in order to shape your dwelling according to your heart's content. A House Blessing is just what you and your home need in order for you both to feel right again! And you can certainly accomplish that, but you have to *want* to. You have to intend that it be so. Many of the spaces we exist in on a daily basis don't take our input or respond to us; enjoy the freedom of a space where *you* set the agenda.

INTENTION

Every day we have a chance to re-create life,
for ourselves and others, reshaping our energies
with the thoughts we think ... Bless the house in which
you wake, and the people who also sleep there.
Bless your city and your country and your world.
Bless everyone you will meet today.
—Marianne Williamson

The definition of intention is this: "An act or instance of determining mentally upon some action or result. A determination to act in a certain way." Intention consciously aims our thoughts and feelings toward what we seek. It is an awesome thing. Science has shown that the mere formulation of an intention sets off the neural synapses in your brain—charges it, if you will. This is literally mind over matter and the first step toward achieving your goal. All action requires an intention. We can't just summon up random energy. We don't know what we will get. And if we don't set our intentions, we lose control of the circumstances of our life. Lacking intention, we can stray, without meaning to, from the path of our vision. But with it, all the forces of the universe can align to make even the seemingly impossible possible. Intention backed by commitment, conscientious attention, and focused energy makes it so.

Dr. Larry Dossey wrote in *Healing Words: The Power of Prayer and the Practice of Medicine,* "Research into quantum mechanics has shown that the act of observing reality creates it. Attempting to observe something causes it to appear out of the nothing." According to Lynne McTaggart, founder of The Intention Project and author of *The Intention Experiment,* "Living consciousness is somehow the influence that turns the possibility of something into something real. The most essential ingredient in creating our universe is the consciousness that observes it. The mind's ability to affect the physical world could be augmented through practice. Intention is a learned skill."

Since intentions are so powerful, it is crucial that they be well conceived from our deepest, most authentic desires and requirements. When we express our intentions, we had better really mean it. This is imperative, for as the saying goes, "You have to be careful of what you wish for, because you will get it." This is the Law of Attraction. Energy goes where you send it.

All action requires an intention. Your intention with a House Blessing is the purpose, your desired outcome: the creation of a warm, welcoming, comfortable, and safe home for you and yours. By the same token, all intentional actions need attention. Attention means staying present, purposeful, and determined in your pursuit of what is needed, starting with having a plan for what to do and how to do it. Paying attention to all the details that make it possible to create the energy you want is what will cause that energy to manifest. In other words, you gotta do the work! You can't cheat or take shortcuts. What would be the point?

Years ago I held a Winter Solstice ceremony on the dock of the South Street Seaport in Manhattan. It is customary to light fires at the solstice, but that's not possible on a landmarked antique wooden dock. So I brought fifty-two battery-operated lanterns to place along the edges of the pier in parallel formation to create a visual path leading to the ceremonial circle. As we were setting up, my intern confessed that we were one short and maintained that it wouldn't matter, because no one would know.

Wrong! I would know. Fifty-two is an intentional number representing the weeks in a year. It means something. There is no point in having fifty-one. And even though the people in attendance wouldn't know in a conscious way, the energy would not resonate the intention subliminally to participants if its source was off.

Your intentions are the foundation of everything you hope to achieve by blessing your house. The ceremony will activate your intentions and your attentive actions will express your vision and make it real. The strength of your intentions is what empowers you to bless your home in the most beneficent manner by filling it with an ambience that radiates your deepest loving attentions and provides the perfect home environment for you.

"Okay. But how do I know how to actually accomplish that?"

EMPOWERMENT

You can accomplish this, because this is your house. No one knows it as you do. Your life is centered there. Remember, you are the expert on you. And don't worry. You can't do it wrong! There is no such thing as a bad blessing. A bad blessing is an oxymoron. A blessing is good and effective as long as it is created and performed with sincere loving intention and careful, respectful attention. Blessing your house will imprint it with your most heartfelt intentions and it is thus transformed.

Love begins at home, and it is not how much we do...
but how much love we put in that action.
—Mother Teresa

There is no one-size-fits-all House Blessing ritual. A ritual created from a recipe book is about as likely to heal us—or hurt us—as following the medical protocol prescribed for someone else is likely to cure us. A blessing ceremony that speaks directly to your particular situation, the members of your household, your belief systems, your aesthetics, and your heartfelt hopes and dreams is just what your space needs.

Despite this, it is commonly believed that Blessings are only to be dispensed from on high by deities and those who are officially ordained. Conventional wisdom says that only ministers, rabbis, priest/esses, imams, sadhus, medicine wo/men, shamans, or gurus are deemed holy enough to design, direct, or officiate at ceremonies of import. While you can certainly seek out a professional such as a clergy member or spiritual practitioner to bless your house, think how much more personal and meaningful your Blessing ritual would be if you were to do it yourself. You are the authority when it comes to living in your home. You know what the energy that surrounds you feels like. And you know how you would like it to feel. So who can better express the depth of your emotions and the fervency of your intentions besides you? You have the key to your home and your domestic desires and requirements are the keys to creating your House Blessing ceremony.

There is a concept in the Ifa religion of the West African Yoruba culture, one of the original sources of the spiritual traditions practiced throughout the African Diaspora in the Caribbean and South America, that "You crown your own head." This means that you make your own life happen, that the response-ability for what transpires rests with each of us. This emphasis on personal power is not isolating individualism. Rather, it is empowering and liberating, leaving you free to trust your own inner voice and to act upon the wisdom of your insights and intentions.

> You have to participate relentlessly
> in the manifestation of your own blessings.
> —Elizabeth Gilbert, *Eat, Pray, Love*

Don't abdicate your spiritual sovereignty. You have within you the wisdom and the emotional resources based on your own unique life experiences to create the most perfect and personally relevant ceremony for your own private space. Your Blessing ritual will be guided by your vision for your home. Claim your Blessing and make it your own. Your Blessing will express your intentions, project your personal desires and beliefs, and reflect the attention and energy you put into the ceremony that you create. You hold that power. You hold the keys.

Ritual is about inclusion. Anything is appropriate as long as it is perfect—that is to say, authentic—well-intentioned, well-conceived, and truly heartfelt. Blessing something or someone is basically a way to dispense goodness, like spreading frosting on a cake. A blessing, like any holy endeavor, is one that begins with a sincere intention; that is acted upon with avid, unwavering attention and commitment; and that is practiced with fervent dedication, love, and piety. A personalized House Blessing designed and performed by you will serve to establish a spirit-filled, energetically charged atmosphere in your home that is deeply meaningful, incredibly powerful, and always perfect.

Keep reading, and in the following chapters you will discover everything you need to know in order to bless your own house with the utmost authority and aplomb. Herein are detailed lists of cleansing and blessing agents along with descriptions, benefits, and explanations of how and when to use them (of course the choice of *what* to use is up to you). There are sample scripts and suggested sequences for House Blessing rituals along with selections of folk wisdom, global prayers, and blessings from many spiritual paths to spur your imagination. These traditional sayings and practices can be used as is in your ceremony however you like, or, ideally, they may inspire you to compose your own special personally relevant blessings.

Remember, there are no rules! No recipes, no prescriptions, no instruction manuals, no precise formulas to follow when planning and performing a Blessing ritual. There are only your own intuition, your best intentions, and your conscientious attention. This does not, however, mean that anything goes. Just as in life, everything matters. This is the bottom line of response-ability. Your intentions have to be perfectly pure and your attention to the details of the process has to be focused and disciplined, in exact alignment with your intentions. The quality of your engagement needs to be really right—not according to the standards of anyone else, but only according to your own inner truth. The only thing you can do wrong in a ritual is to not pay attention to your true intentions. As my Gramma used to say in her thick Yiddish accent while she was baking, "A leetle butta. A leetle shuga, vat could be bad?" What, indeed, could be bad about a blessing?

My longtime friend Paul is an excellent role model in this regard. Nearly four decades ago I facilitated a wonderful community ritual in the park across the street from my loft. "Ceremony to Save the Last Sycamore" took place on May Day, the traditional time to honor green growth. We spent the entire day connecting this poor scraggly dying tree with colorful twine to all of the living trees and bushes in this four-acre public space, creating a gigantic web of care and concern.

At dusk we dug a hole at the foot of the ailing tree and then we separated, each one of us going home to fetch a perfect small healing item to bury in its roots as a blessing for its healing. Paul, my downstairs neighbor, asked me if he could bring sugar to the Blessing ritual. Taken aback, I thought, "sugar? *Sugar??*" But I said, "Sure, why not?"

Well, Paul showed up with his sugar in a beautiful antique Limoges sugar bowl. Using a well-shined engraved silver spoon, he sprinkled the sparkly white granules all around the perimeter of the ceremonial ground as reverentially as if he were offering incense at the Vatican, copal at an Aztec temple, or corn pollen at a Navajo ceremonial. Watching Paul, the sweetest guy I knew, dispense delicious loving blessings in such a deeply authentic manner moved me to tears. And the ailing sycamore tree did not die.

"Yes, that's a nice story, but how will *I* know how to actually do a blessing?" you inquire.

There are any number of ways that you can bless your home. The techniques might vary, but the idea is always the same—to claim and consecrate your home as yours by whatever means seem appropriate to you. As always, the quality of the attention that you pay to creating your blessings will reflect the purity of your intention. There are no particular words to say, nor incense to light. The special words are the ones that you want to hear and the herbs are the ones that you want to smell. This is your venture, your ritual, your room, your headquarters, your home. Your blessing can be anything that you want it to be—as long as it is meaningful to you.

Don't worry about getting it right. There is no "right" except what you choose to do. Trust your heart of hearts and your own deepest knowing that you will use exactly the right elements and words to express and further your dreams and plans. Only you know what resonates with your ideas. What are your goals and intentions? What speaks to you about these? It is that deep personal resonance that makes a blessing so powerful. Try creating a blessings journal and filling it with all the inspiration that speaks to you.

A client of mine once told me that for as long as she could remember, she had a burning desire to move to San Francisco, but she never acted on it. I suggested that she create an altar with images of San Francisco—pictures, maps, small toys and models symbolizing the cable cars, Fisherman's Wharf, Chinatown, etc. She even drew her idea of a perfect San Francisco house. This was the stage set where she performed her daily San Francisco Dream House Blessing. She finally made her move just six months after she set up her altar.

As for what words to say, just open your mouth and let them flow in a stream of consciousness. Or read a favorite quote. Or recite a favorite prayer. Or walk through your space and sing to it, a Blessing serenade. Or, or, or, or. You choose! In the end it is your intention and the attention you put toward expressing it that is important. I have every confidence that your Blessing will be beautiful and powerful, and precisely what you need it to be. Best blessings on your Blessing.

Find joy in everything you choose to do.
Every job, relationship, home . . .
it's your responsibility to love it or change it.
—Chuck Palahniuk, American novelist and
freelance journalist

This is your home.
It can be any way you want it to be.

Blessing is the lifeblood throbbing
through the universe.

—Brother David Steindl-Rast
99 Blessings: An Invitation to Life

CHAPTER 4

Welcome Home

Global House Blessing Ceremonies are as old as houses themselves. Historically, they have begun before there is even a house, starting with the blessings of the earth itself for permission to build on it. There are infinite ways to cleanse and bless the energy of an abode, during construction, when first moving in, or at any later date when the need arises. Blessings of the ground in gratitude before it is first broken. Blessings of the foundation for strength and stability. Blessings of the support beams, of the first stone or brick laid for strength and durability. And continuing with each step of the construction process until the house is completed. Blessings of the roof for weather protection. Blessings of the door for both welcome and security. Blessings of the façade for safekeeping, luck, and good fortune. Blessings of the hearth for warmth, nurturing spirit, and conviviality.

Here are just a few examples of traditions around sanctifying everything from the plot of land to the building stones in different cultures around the world. If particular elements of these practices speak to you, feel free to incorporate them into a House Blessing that you design. Or use them as inspiration to spark your own creative approach to consecrating your home in a very personal way.

GROUNDING

The Tlingit, Haida, and Tsimshian people of the Pacific Northwest of the United States believe that everything has a spirit, so before they begin construction of a house, they offer chants and dances of thanksgiving to Mother Earth and the ground on which they will build, as well as to the cedar trees in gratitude for their sacrifice in providing the poles for the new structure.

The Kikuyu people of Kenya also perform Blessing rituals before commencing a building project. A goat is sacrificed to the earth where the ancestors dwell, for good luck. The sacrificial blood is sprinkled on the ground of the site and also on the tools and conveyances that will be used in the construction. It was the tradition in Mykonos, Greece that the blood of a rooster must flow fresh onto the earth at the site where a new home is to be built, an offering that ensures protection for all who will eventually enter. In India, milk, spices, and incense are offered to purify the land and the building crew is given traditional gifts of fruits and chocolates.

These earth-honoring rituals in preparation for building a structure on the land have continued to this day. Ground Breaking ceremonies are quite common in many places around the world. Prayers for protection and success usually precede the actual breaking of the ground, which is then accomplished by a chosen luminary who has the honor of digging the first shovelful of dirt.

Recently an archaeological expedition in Sardis, an ancient city in modern-day Turkey, unearthed a cache of eggs in a clay pot that had been buried under the dirt floor of a Roman house almost two thousand years ago, most likely as part of a purification ritual. According to Nick Cahill, the director of the dig, "Burying items in homes as a ritual isn't itself an unusual practice; it's a common tradition throughout the Mediterranean and Near East." In Greece you find a lot of these types of deposits, where something was put in the walls as a dedication.

Many ceramic bowls inscribed with blessings in Judeo-Aramaic languages have been found buried under the foundation of houses in ancient Babylonia, Mesopotamia, and Iraq, dating from AD 200 to AD 800. These incantation bowls, also known as devil bowls and demon traps, are protective charms meant to trap any bad spirits and safeguard the building and its residents from bad energy and evildoers. It is an age-old Andean custom before building a house in Bolivia to bury a llama fetus in the earth beneath the foundation to help give the owners good fortune. Mummified llama fetuses are still sold in the markets there for this purpose.

BUILDING

When constructing a masonry edifice, be it a pyramid, a cathedral, or a house, the first stone laid has special significance, since all further stones or bricks will be placed adjacent to it or on top of it, thus determining the shape and strength of the entire structure. Thus, the foundation stone has long been treated as a ceremonial building block that represents the birth of the building and is blessed with offerings of grain, oil, and wine, and in ancient times with animal and, sometimes, human sacrifice to ensure the stability of the building. The stone blocks often had a hollowed-out indentation to hold a time capsule or a vial of wine in honor of this auspicious new beginning.

The setting of the foundation stone in Malaysia is celebrated in a ritual by Brahmin or Lama priests offering flowers, by masons or by carpenters with sacrificial chickens or a lamb, or by the youngest son of the owner of the building, who beats on the stone with a hammer to create a vibration to connect the stone with the positive energies of the cosmos. In Sri Lanka, the foundation stone is a special concrete stone with a cavity that is filled with precious metals and grains. Speckles of copper, bronze, gold, silver, precious stones, grains, and sacred objects are included to bring positive energy to the new house.

Over time and with the advent of modern metal-and-glass skyscrapers, foundation stone rituals have morphed into celebrations of the cornerstone. When construction is finished, the cornerstone is engraved with the names of the architect and the builder and the dates of construction and completion. It is then set into the façade of the building with much protective pomp and circumstance, every bit a contemporary lucky talisman. The Order of Masons offers Foundation Stone ceremonies to be held at building sites of all kinds.

RAISING THE BEAMS

Once the land and material have been consecrated, there are other rituals around the building materials as they come together. In Sumatra the first two pillars are connected by a horizontal beam to each other, then raised into place while verses from the Quran are recited. When the building is finished these will form the main room of the house. If this important part of the construction takes place smoothly, the house building can then be continued with good luck. Throughout Southeast Asia, after the support beams are installed and before roofing starts, a bunch of flowers is tied at one end of the ridge, and strips of red fabric are hung between the pillars like prayer flags. In Java, black and white cloths are added to the red. Several offerings such as coconuts, bananas, and plants are also tied to the king post as a feast to the good spirits of the house. In ancient China, the ridgepole of a new structure was smeared with chicken blood, as a substitute offering for human blood, in hopes of fooling the deities.

In Europe the setting of the ridge beams in place was consecrated by sprinkling wine on the completed work, after which the workers celebrated by drinking the rest of the wine. It is speculated that the ritual of ridge beam setting is a result of the technical inability of the traditional architects and craftsmen to build a structure that was strong enough to stand stable against strong storms and earthquakes. So a ceremony was performed to petition the spirit powers for strength and stability of the structure and favorable weather.

RAISING THE ROOF

The Gwana people of Ethiopia build edifices to house ancestral spirits. These are similar to human dwellings, but smaller. The roofs are hung with the first fruits of corn, or offerings such as coconuts, bananas, and plants are tied to the king post as a feast to entice the good spirits of the house, and sorghum and hunting paraphernalia are placed on the roof to be blessed by the spirits residing in these ceremonial houses. Since imperial times in Japan, an architectural ritual called *muneage*, which means roof raising, has been celebrated when the roof of a structure has been installed. An altar is placed on the roof and a Shinto ceremony involving flowers, invocations, and rice, offered in gratitude for the successful construction of a protective roof overhead, is performed there.

Communities often play a key supportive role worldwide in creating the proper space. Barns are one obvious example—crucial for a farmer's success, but too big to be built by one or a few people. Raising a barn or a church, a school or a Habitat for Humanity house requires many hands. Barn raisings, known as raising or rearing bees in the United Kingdom, are collective community actions where neighbors join together en masse to build barns or homes for each other in reciprocal mutual support. This tradition is still practiced among Amish and Old Order Mennonites in the Midwest of the United States and Canada. Very much in the spirit of Amish barn raisings, Andean villages hold house-roofing rituals known as the *zafacasa* to forge strong social bonds of community and acknowledgement and gratitude of interdependence.

Topping out, sometimes called topping off, is a ritual celebrated upon the completion of a building. When an edifice has reached its intended height it is topped with a flag or a tree. This practice can be traced to the seventh century AD Scandinavian tradition of hoisting an evergreen tree to the top of a newly built house to celebrate the end of construction. The tree, symbolizing the tree of life, served as a blessing of fertility and long life to the newlywed couple who would inhabit the house. Teutonic tribes may have used these ceremonial trees to appease the tree spirits for having killed trees for lumber. Germans living in the Black Forest observed this Christmas tree custom in honor of the nativity of Jesus Christ, and to this day, evergreen trees top off nearly every new structure in Germany. The Swiss also claim to have started the practice of displaying a fir tree to celebrate topping out.

The custom of putting a tree on top of a newly completed structure traveled with northern European immigrant builders to their new homes. Today, topping-off ceremonies are popular and often well publicized among steelworkers on construction sites across the urban world. Typically, the final beam installed on the top of a skyscraper is painted white and signed by the entire crew, after which glasses are lifted in celebration as many as one hundred stories in the sky.

RAISING THE SPIRITS

The Navajo consecrate a new dwelling, or *hogan*, by marking the four sacred directions with cornmeal, or sometimes with corn pollen, charcoal, ashes, or other substances. Cornmeal symbolizes life and success along the road, often appearing in ceremonies. These marks are applied inside the hogan at the highest part that can be reached, just as the Holy People, First Man and First Woman, did in the Navajo creation myth. This blessing also ensures that the hogan is purified of any influences that might be considered taboo.

When the construction of a native Hawaiian's home is complete, they may invite the local *kahu* or spiritual leader to bless it by sprinkling water and cleansing salt around the perimeter of the house to symbolically wrap it with protection. It is also very common to decorate the new house with colors and other safeguarding symbols as a protective shield.

In Thailand, monks bless new houses by using white paste to mark all the doors to ward off evil spirits. People in Morocco, Egypt, and many parts of North Africa have long applied a band of cobalt blue around all windows, doors, and shutters with a mineral substance, which is the same bluing that is added to laundry detergent to clean clothes. The cleansing powder assures protection from tainted energy. The Mexican artist Frida Kahlo painted her entire home, which she named *Casa Azul* or Blue House, with the same stuff, as a prescription to keep the devil away.

It is customary in the American South to paint the ceiling of the front porch, doors, windows, and shutters with paint called "haint blue." This practice stems from the Gullah tradition of the descendants of the slaves in the Low Country of South Carolina and Georgia that was influenced by their African roots. *Haint* means "haunt." The belief is that since ghosts, the haint spirits, are not able to cross water, they will be scared away by so much blue. It's common for houses and barns in Pennsylvania Dutch and Pennsylvania German country to sport brightly painted hex signs. The derivation of these paintings stems back to pre-Christian Alpine German symbols for protection. *Hex* means "witch" in Old German.

After the house itself is completed, people everywhere create another layer of protection by placing guardian figures and lucky plants around the home. Ceramic gnomes are common garden figures in Europe and North America. Folklore tells us that gnomes are friendly creatures who bring good luck and keep a house safe from danger. They sit in the garden to keep watch. Another popular protective garden feature is the Gazing Mirror, a spherical mirror made of colored glass that rests upon a stand or sits on the grass. Gazing Mirrors work to avert the gaze of ill fortune from the home.

They are also known as witches balls, because they ward off the evil eye.

DOORWAYS

The doorway of any domicile is a magical portal that invites you to enter a new environment, a new perspective, a new experience, a new attitude, and the possibility of a new way of life. A single step takes you from one reality into another—from outside to inside, from dark to light, from public to private, and vice versa. When you open the door and cross the threshold of your new home for the first time on the day that you move in, you are embarking on a life-changing opportunity for a clean start and a new adventure in living, not so unlike Neil Armstrong's fateful footfall on the moon. This simple one-step movement is a sacred act of faith and hope and optimistic determination tinged with an underlying trepidation of the unfamiliar. Such an auspicious undertaking calls for intentional acts of blessing to ensure that the door of your new place will assure a safe and supportive environment in which to live, grow, and thrive. This has always been so.

Since doors have such spiritual significance, people everywhere have regarded them as sacred. According to feng shui, the Chinese philosophical system of arranging one's surroundings to be in alignment and harmony with the natural world, the door is the most important part of an edifice. Doors are considered to be the mouth of the house and are called the "Mouth of Chi." Chi is energy. In China, doors are often painted red, the color of power, energy, and chi. Energy can be positive or negative, and the mouth can swallow it or spit it out. The door to your new home opens to welcome fortune in and closes like armor for safekeeping against danger. Red flowers in window boxes also offer powerful protection. Geraniums are especially popular across Europe for this purpose.

Because they can open and shut, doorways and windows are thought to be vulnerable to invasion by unwanted evil energy entering the space. So folks everywhere hang amulets and charms above or around their doors as petitions to whatever power they believe in for blessings of favored beginnings, good fortune, and freedom from harm. These talismans work as guardians that create a virtual checkpoint and impenetrable boundary.

The biblical Book of Exodus tells that the ancient Israelites were instructed by God to slaughter a lamb and mark their doors with its blood. Houses with these marks would be passed over and not suffer the loss of their children in the plagues. Some Muslims inscribe the name of Allah and verses of the Koran over their doors and windows for protection. Devout Catholics bless their homes by writing the initials of the three kings—C + M + B—above the doors of their houses during the Christmas season using chalk that has been blessed in the church for this use.

Jews everywhere affix mezuzahs on the doorposts of their homes, as per a biblical commandment: "Write the words of God on the gates and doorposts of your house." The mezuzah is a decorative case, usually made of metal, that contains a rolled parchment scroll inscribed with Hebrew prayers and verses. Those who hang them are thought to be protected from evil and destructive forces. *Nazars*, glass charms in the shape of an eye, are hung above doorways in Greece and Turkey to ward off the evil eye. The evil eye is defeated in Arabic and Berber culture by attaching a *hamsa* on the door. These are talismans shaped like a human palm with a sees-all eye symbol in the center. In Morocco they are called "Hands of Fatima."

A Japanese Shinto belief is that the *ofuda*, a decorated amulet made of wood, paper, cloth, or metal attached to the door, is a powerful protection from disease for those who dwell inside. *Palaspas* are decorative palm fronds sold in the Philippines on Palm Sunday. They are blessed by a priest and then hung over the doors of homes. They serve as a talisman to ward off evil. Ancient Egyptians hung bundles of cinnamon sticks above the door to protect and sanctify the entrance area. It is a Celtic custom to hang wreaths made of rosemary or woven rowan branches tied into cross shapes and wrapped in red thread to safeguard the house and family.

> Rowan tree, red thread,
> holds the witches all in dread.
> —Celtic Rhyme

Attaching bouquets of garlic to doors for protection from ghoulies and ghosties and blood-sucking vampires is common across the planet. Ancient Egyptians thought that the vampirelike ghosts that suck the breath out of their sleeping children were repelled by garlic at the entranceway. Romanians believe that vampires are afraid of garlic, so they smear a paste of it on the doors and windows of their homes as well as the gates of their farms and on the horns of their bulls. Serbians to this day hang braids of garlic bulbs on the door to scare away vampires. During the witch-burning times in Europe when evil spirits were thought to be on the loose, it became a

popular style to wear necklaces made of garlic cloves to
ward off demons and protect one's vulnerable throat.

Feng shui practice suggests several good luck charms
to put at the front door. A *bagua* mirror placed above the
doorframe welcomes good fortune and harmony to a home
and all who enter. It also blocks entrance to any negative
chi. Bamboo flutes are symbols of strength and support.
Hanging such a flute on the door with the mouthpiece
facing up will secure a home from any negative forces.
Wind bells are used in China to protect homes. The
Japanese hang glass bells called *ūrin* to attract good luck,
and today, glass, metal, wood, and ceramic wind chimes are
very popular throughout Europe and the United States for
their soothing sound, which creates good vibes.

In Portugal and in the large Portuguese community in
Newark, New Jersey, mirrors are mounted outside above
the doors and windows of a house to reflect and repel any
harmful energy trying to get in. Horseshoes are hung over
doorways in many cultures. They are usually placed above
the door with the legs up, which creates a vessel to hold the
good luck for the residents of this home. It is also common to
display them with the legs pointing down so that good luck
will flow upon all who come and go through this doorway.
In the West of the United States folks hang arrowheads as a

deterrent against burglary. Catholics sometimes hang a holy water font next to the door, while it is customary in the Dominican Republic to hang bread over the door to ensure that food will never be scarce.

THE THRESHOLD

Beneath the door is the threshold, the psychic borderline that separates the outside realms from the inside, the domestic scene from the natural world. In old Holland it was taboo to actually step on the threshold, or *drempel*, because the devil was said to be asleep beneath it and the sound of a footstep would wake him and cause him to raise hell. This belief gave birth to the tradition of the groom carrying his bride over the threshold of their new home after the wedding, a sacred crossing from one reality to another.

Houses are often blessed at the first crossing of the threshold even before moving in. A Hindu rite or *Puja* is performed for the threshold in honor of the deities who reside there and guard the owner by refusing entrance to any evil forces. A Vastu Puja is performed before stepping into the house to invite goodness to enter the space. On this day the owners and family members enter the new house at a carefully chosen auspicious time and in a particular order: The wife steps across the threshold with her right foot, carrying a pot full of water. Following is her husband, bearing an image of the gods. Then the children enter, carrying groceries that represent prosperity. And finally, other relatives step in. In addition to the first crossing, Hindus celebrate three additional House-warming ceremonies: When the house is constructed on a newly selected land. On entering into the house after a stay abroad or elsewhere. When entering into a resold house and after the house is repaired or renovated due to the damage caused by natural or unnatural calamities.

In Laos and Thailand a family performs a *Sen Wai Jour Teen* ceremony before moving into a new home as a way to make their presence known. They politely inform the spirits that they will be occupying the house from now on, and humbly request their divine guardianship. Blessings of food, flowers, and incense sticks are offered to appease any wandering ghosts so that they will bring good luck to the family and not make trouble.

Each new dwelling, or hogan, that is built must be blessed, according to the Navajo way. The Navajo House Blessing ceremony is called *hooghan da ashdlisigil* in the Navajo language and is performed to benefit both the inhabitants and the hogan itself with protection and blessings for peace. This ritual is a way to feed the house and show it proper respect as a living being so as to prevent structural damage and soothe the hogan's loneliness, which can attract evil spirits if not healed. Blessings are offered to promote peace, harmony, good luck, and well-being and to prevent hardship, wind and fire destruction, illness, bad dreams, and general misfortune for those whose lives the hogan shelters. Smudging, the burning of bundles of dried plants such as tobacco, sage, juniper, cedar, copal, yerba santa, and palo santo is a common Blessing among many Native Peoples of the Americas. This holy smoke dispels negative energy and promotes healing. The ascending smoke carries the prayers of the worshiper to the Creator. Before moving, in the Caribbean, folks roll a burning coconut along the floor to rid the space of bad spirits.

In Russia and Portugal, people always send a cat inside a new house or apartment before they actually move in. The cat will sniff out and scare away any evil entities. The Tamils who live in the far south of India bless a new house by inviting a cow to walk through every room of the house first to bring good fortune to the household. All gods are believed to reside in the cow, so it is decorated and worshiped with flowers, turmeric, and *kumkum*, a pigment made of turmeric. The cow and her calf are then taken to all the rooms. After the bovine blessings, some of the cow's milk is boiled in the kitchen, to symbolically light the domestic flame. This description by David Sun appeared in Singapore's *The New Paper* in 2014:

> "It was a strange sight that greeted residents at Eight Courtyards condominium in Canberra Drive when a cow and calf were led through the grounds. A man with gloves, a bucket and trash bags followed closely behind the animals, just in case the animals defecated in public. The animals squeezed into a lift and went up to the fourteenth story of one of the blocks, where the Thiagarajen family was waiting expectantly. The family had just moved into their new home and the animals were there to do a House Blessing. Sri Vanitha, thirty-five, was delighted at the arrival of her 'guests' to her newly renovated home. She was even more happy to see them dropping feces and spraying urine all over the living room floor. She said: 'It's the first time in my house and I'm very contented. It is a blessing.'"

Customs of many cultures suggest bringing certain items into a new abode in order to appease the spirits. The Thai celebrate a ritual called *Keun Ban Mai*, which means "going up into a new house." This is a two-part ritual. First, the family arrives at the appointed auspicious time along with their furniture, and carrying symbols of Buddha, food, and money to ensure a prosperous future in the house. This is followed by a *Sai Seen*, "Holy Thread ceremony," in which a length of string is connected to the door and led from the entranceway to the house Buddha, wound around the wrists of the family, and then threaded through the hands of the monks gathered in prayer. Their chanting vibrates through the strings and sets off charged energy meant to protect the house and the family.

People in India are also careful about choosing an astrologically appropriate day and time to cross the threshold of their new home for the first time. In order to do so, they consult a priest who consults astrology charts to work out the perfect horoscope for their move-in date. They invite relatives and friends to witness the auspicious occasion and join in the blessings and festivities, after which the family members stay in the house for a few days, even if it is still unfurnished, so that they can absorb the optimistic energies that were generated by the warm company and the Cleansing and Blessing rituals performed.

MOVING DAY

And now, finally, after all the many preparatory rituals, it is time to actually move in, which always calls for a party and celebratory rites. In China, it is customary to throw a House Leaving party for friends and neighbors just before moving into the new home. Fireworks are set off. And then, again, as they enter their new digs accompanied by a retinue of well-wishers, there is another pyrotechnic display. A fellow New Yorker advocates for this farewell ritual, "Always leave a can of beans in the pantry of an apartment you are leaving for the next tenant, because you never know when tough times will hit." While he hopes he'll never have to use the beans he gave away, he believes that leaving a can of beans will bring good luck to the new tenant as well as to himself.

It is very common for people everywhere who are moving out of their old home to disassemble their altars; remove their mezuzahs, icons, religious statuary, and other spiritual installations, and sometimes even their plantings; and take them into their new abode. In this way the sanctity of one dwelling space is transferred to another, always keeping the spiritual connection to home alive wherever it might be. This act is the reverse of a housewarming, rather it is a house cooling, as it were. A once obscure practice that has gained a certain popularity among contemporary house sellers is to bury a statue of Saint Joseph upside down in the dirt of their yard in the belief that he will move heaven and earth on their behalf to achieve a sale. That accomplished, he is exhumed and placed in a prime spot on the mantle of the new home.

When moving into a new house, Thai people bring rice, water, and a knife. Rice and water are brought as wishes for a good, prosperous life, and the knife is for protection from evil spirits. In many Asian societies, a new house ritual involves sprinkling rice grains in all the rooms in the house for assurance of plenty to eat. Pineapples are a widely popular symbol of hospitality and good luck. Hokkien people of China buy the biggest ripe pineapple in the market and, with the crown intact, roll it into the house and around the floors of each room. Occasionally, the pineapple is smashed on the floor of a new house, then the door is quickly closed and the bits and pieces are left around for a few days to impart sweet blessings.

Various practical items are also offered as good-luck moving gifts. In Korea people organize parties for new homes known as *jibdeuli*. The guests usually bring rolls of toilet paper and some detergent, as they are considered to be symbols of prosperity, since they were once too expensive for many families to afford. Brooms are popular housewarming gifts in Europe. This is important, because bringing a broom from an old house is dangerous, as it is filled with old troubles. A new broom will keep the house clean and sweep away evil spirits bringing bad luck. Baskets, too, are double-duty housewarming presents. They are, of course, handy receptacles, but in addition are thought to catch and hold the stress and worries of the residents.

Some Chinese attach great significance to bringing a bamboo pole into the house. The joints on bamboo ascend one above another, which symbolizes the wish for growth, progress, and attainment in life, which makes them an appropriate blessing present. It is also considered a good-luck practice to bring an orange or tangerine tree into the home. This practice is significant, because the Chinese words for orange and luck sound very similar.

HOUSEWARMING

The ultimate Housewarming ceremony is to actually bring light and warmth into an empty, dark place. Chinese people enter the empty house carrying small stoves filled with burning charcoal. The fiery vessels are placed in every corner of every room to smoke out any negative energy and to make sure the hostile spirits have no place to hide. Then, before moving furniture and other belongings into the house, they shine a light in every corner, closet, and drawer to let any lingering spirits know that it is time for them to leave and show them the way to exit the premises. The People of the Pacific Northwest Coast practice a "lighting-up" of a house ceremony by carrying a candle through the entire house to push light into every crevice and corner.

In many traditions, candles are burned in prayer offerings, in blessings, and also in celebration. Lighting candles on the first night in a new home is a symbolic casting-off of the dark, the dangerous, and the hidden negative forces that will no longer be able to hide in the shadows. Lighting a fire in the fireplace when moving in is a warming tradition kept alive since medieval times. Fire is a potent symbol for strength, purity, and positive power. As it burns away stagnant energy and lurking spirits, it illuminates and consecrates new, optimistic beginnings.

Food plays a central role in the spiritual warming of new homes everywhere. Food represents life, nurturing, health, pleasure, conviviality, family, community—everything that a good home offers. Buddhists in Nepal bless homes in a ceremony that includes one whole red fish, rice, sake, and rock salt. In Jewish and Russian custom, guests bring bread, wine, sugar, and salt when they visit someone's new home. A Housewarming gift of bread is common throughout the western world and is given to ensure that the family will always have enough food to eat. Wine represents always having enough to drink, an abundance of joy and prosperity, and plenty of occasions to celebrate. Wine is also used as a sacrament. Salt symbolizes the blood, sweat, and tears of life. And sugar and honey are blessings for sweet fortune.

> Abounding in food, abounding in milk,
> with firm foundation set on the earth,
> receptacle of every nourishing thing,
> do no harm, O House,
> to those who receive you.
> —Hindu House Blessing

Since the Middle Ages, when construction of a new home is finished, the French throw a traditional party called the *pendre la crémaillère*, literally meaning "to hang the chimney hook." This hook, called a *trammel*, was used to hang cauldrons over the fire. It was the last thing installed in the house, meaning that now cooking would be possible. Everyone who has taken part in the building of the house is invited to eat dinner as a gesture of thanks. The freshly ignited fire along with the expressed gratitude and conviviality literally and symbolically warm the new house. In some parts of the United States, people light the oven in their new home for the first time and bake a cake, which is then brought to their new neighbors to introduce themselves.

The United States is home to people of all cultures. We all carry childhood memories of family traditions and stories of the old-world customs of our forebearers. We also have unlimited access to information and images of ceremonies and celebrations practiced around the world. From this eclectic treasure chest we can each create our own personally relevant rituals to consecrate our own home. What did you do to celebrate/sanctify the day you moved into your home?

A few years ago, the *New York Times* posted a story about House Blessings on their Facebook page and asked readers how they went about blessing their new homes. Here are some of the answers:

- I used to burn a smudge stick in a new apartment for good luck. But after my husband and I bought a house twelve years ago, something better happened quite by accident: Our niece, a toddler, ran laughing through all the empty rooms. I couldn't think of a better blessing.

- We use a three-step process: first, salt is put in all the corners to dispel bad spirits; next, candy is placed around the house to bring in sweetness; lastly, sage and saltwater are used to cleanse and purify the space, calling in blessing and happiness.

- I sprinkle salt (to soak up old tears) and rosewater (to purify) on all the doorsteps.

- We're buying a new house soon...and while we don't try to evict old auras, we do search out good ones. ALSO we factor in new bathrooms into the price. I WILL NOT set foot in someone's old bathtub. NO WAY.

- A few years ago, my boyfriend severed a vein and tendon in his index finger while helping me move into a new apartment. I'm normally a pretty logical person, but I smudged like crazy after that. (I did take him to the emergency room to get stitched up first.) Say what you will, but I felt better, everybody comments on how welcoming the place is, and nobody's gotten hurt there since.

- I repaint every wall. I don't care if it was just done. A fresh coat of paint is a personal thing.

- Chinese takeout and a bottle of wine on the floor before I even start to unpack.

- I'm from the South. It's tradition to hang a horseshoe, with its U shape up, over the front door. It catches good luck.

- I was always told to leave a broom behind at the residence you were leaving. When the new people moved in, they were to use that broom to sweep the apartment or house, then throw that broom away, I suppose along with whatever juju was attached to the former residents.

- I throw coins in first before entering for the first time. Just like throwing coins in the fountain, then I make a wish.

- We ate twelve grapes, had thirteen golden coins in a red sack during dinner, broomed from the inside to the outside, threw a glass of water (well, just the water), and lit all the lights in the house to attract light and energy.

- The best "ritual" I ever had was entirely unplanned and of the best sort: a bluebird lighted on the crepe myrtle outside the kitchen window on my first day in my new house and sat there preening for several minutes as though he owned the place. I figured it was an omen: "the bluebird of happiness."

- We have a menorah, Japanese New Year wreath, and religious idols and crucifixes on our threshold. We have all religions covered and more!!

- We do it in every room in the house on the first night.

- Smudged each room, opened the windows wide overnight the first night, placed a ring of ash around the perimeter of the house. Then I walked the land and gave thanks to each of the large trees to let them know there were new caretakers for the land.

- Our family tradition was to bring to a new home some salt (for prosperity), bread (for nurture/health), and a candle (enlightenment). Bring them before moving in. Tiny portions were fine, and we used/ate them later (a practical family).

Home is a name, a word, it is a strong one;
stronger than magician ever spoke,
or spirit ever answered to, in the strongest conjuration.
—Charles Dickens, *Martin Chuzzlewit*

A home is a home is a home.
Cherished everywhere.

At heart, giving a blessing is really quite simple.
We innately know how to do it, precisely because
it comes from the heart, from a sense of
caring and helpfulness.

—Frederic and Mary Ann Brussat
The Blessing Path

CHAPTER 5

Homemade Blessings

Congratulations! Now that you are confident that you have identified your feelings and intentions for your home and given thought to how you will manifest them, you are ready to create and perform your own personalized blessing of your space.

Here is a sample outline for a simple House Blessing ceremony based on some of the Cleansing and Blessing rituals that I have developed over the decades. It is an amalgam of the most common ceremonial practices from around the globe, augmented with lists of suggestions of what to do, what to say, and what to use. These menus offer a mix-and-match selection of appropriate supplies and tools to use, sample texts to read, and alternative ceremonial scenarios. Your blessings can follow these suggestions or they can be spontaneous, letting the energy of the space lead you to express your hopes and dreams as you feel them in the moment.

But first, a note about cultural appropriation:

So much of what we use—food, medicine, material goods, customs, and even words—has come from someplace else. They have been grown, invented, produced, or practiced in other societies. The Web has made the world so much smaller, more accessible, and more interactive so that we are all influenced by each other one way or another, especially here in the United States, where we are privileged to be part of such a glorious mosaic of diverse cultures.

Using something from somewhere else is not in and of itself disrespectful. Burning herbs, for instance, or reciting a blessing or song with respect, appreciation, attribution, and gratitude is honoring that tradition without usurping it. It is decidedly not cool to take on another culture by mimicking it, however. We cannot just put on someone else's tradition as if it were a costume. Nor should we perform sacred rituals that are not from our own heritage unless we have been initiated into their practice. Unfortunately, there are people who do just that, offering sweat lodges, pipe ceremonies, Ayawasca rituals, and so on, earning the ire of the legitimate holders of these traditions.

Thirty-something years ago, I spent time in the Sierra Madre Occidental Mountains in the wilds of Mexico with my shamanic mentor, a Mazatec healer and ritualist. At the end of my stay she blessed me to do my work—*my* work, *not* to carry on her work. I am not a Mazatec and she had her own lineage—daughters, nieces, grand- and great-granddaughters. Plus I don't live in a mud-and-wattle hut in a rainforest, treacherous miles to the nearest town. I am a modern woman living in New York City; thus, I am an authentic urban shaman who creates rituals for my contemporary cosmopolitan community of many cultures. You, too, will find your own work. Be respectful in how you incorporate ancient traditions, and your rituals will vibrate on their own frequency.

HONOR YOUR OWN WISDOM

Despite whatever any expert, teacher, or writer (including me) might tell you to do or how to do it, if it does not resonate with you, if the suggestions are not personally meaningful, do not follow them. This is *your* home. This is *your* life. Do what feels right to you. This is *your* ceremony for *your* space. It is important that the ritual speak to *your* personal needs, intentions, aesthetics, and language. Please feel free to make any additions, subtractions, or changes that feel right to you in order to create *your* own version. I always say, "If the phone rings, answer it. It is for you!" And remember, there can be no wrong blessing.

Your House Blessing ceremony can be done alone or with others. It is best if all the members of the household—kids and pets included—join in, as well as friends, family, neighbors, and roommates, if you so choose—and, of course, if they are willing. Some folks might balk at participating in something unfamiliar to them, but in my experience, people are usually delighted at the prospect of sharing in a special communal experience that will enhance their enjoyment of their homes. When the Home Team collaborates to create a spirited collective energy in your shared domain, everybody benefits from it. The more positive, uplifting intentions you invoke, the better.

A House Blessing ceremony typically proceeds in three stages:

STAGE 1. CLEARING THE ENERGY

- Begin by cleaning the physical space. Sweep, dust, vacuum, and wash everything. Pay special attention to corners and the spaces behind and underneath furniture and cabinets. These dark, hard-to-reach spaces are perfect traps for any residual negativity. Open the windows so that the dirty energy can escape and the breezes can refresh the air inside. This is to physically and spiritually erase the feelings, attitudes, activities, and moods left by previous owners, tenants, builders, and all of their various associates—even previous versions of yourself—in order to open the space for a new chapter of your life.

- Form a procession with all the participants—a spirit conga line, if you will. Walk—or run, skip, jump, dance—around the perimeter of your home on the outside (assuming it is not an apartment) and through each room inside. This is a way to define the boundaries of your physical and spiritual property and to claim it as your own.

- As you move, scare away any intrusive, dark-feeling energy with loud sounds like shouting, singing, whistling, clapping hands. Ringing bells, shaking rattles, or banging on pots and pans works too. Noise chases off bad spirits, which is why people set off fireworks at New Year, to prevent any nasty old energy from entering the incoming year.

- Burn incense (or sage, or cedar, or copal, or frankincense, or juniper, or palo santo, or camphor) to create fragrant purifying smoke to bless with as you parade around and through your place. Spread the smoke with a fan or a feather or your hand or even just your breath, getting it into every corner, closet, and crevice to rout out stinky stale energy. Pay special attention to nooks that can trap disruptive spirits. This ceremonial clearing with smoke is called "smudging," and has been used throughout history, with each culture using locally sourced herbs and resins. Its earliest recorded appearance was in ancient Egypt, as part of religious ceremonies. Smudging with sage, cedar, and sweetgrass has been widely used by Native North Americans for centuries and now the use of sage, especially, has become popular with a wide variety of spiritual folks around the globe. Incense, meanwhile, has been used in liturgical rituals since the early church, and a strong incense culture came to Japan with the import of Buddhism by the Tang monk Ganjin.

STAGE 2.   CHARGING AND BLESSING THE ENERGY

- Once the space has been purified of any negative feelings, it is ready to receive your bountiful blessings for new beginnings. Now is the time to invite in all the beneficent spirits. Lavish your space with love, so that it becomes a gracious receptacle of your sweetest dreams.

- Retrace the path you took to cleanse your house. Bless the outside of the house, the yard, and the ground it stands on by offering gifts to entice the sweet, loving, protective energy. You can scatter cornmeal to bless Mother Earth, like many traditional peoples of North America do. Or toss flower petals or pollen, or sprinkle salt, sugar, glitter, holy water, or any other offering that appeals to you. Plant crystals in your garden. Crystals hold a lot of energy and serve to focus your intentions. Some particularly helpful crystals for attracting luck, protection, and abundance to your home are: green aventurine for luck, jade for luck and prosperity, obsidian for protection, clear quartz for luck and money, and rose quartz for comfort, caring, and warm, loving feelings.

- Bless the perimeters of each room inside and welcome all the protective, lucky, abundant, fruitful spirits to enter and stay in your home and your life. Touch the walls, the doorways, the floors, and the windows as you walk through, anointing them with the burning smoke of sweetgrass, fragrant oils, holy water, caresses, kisses, or your favorite perfume and your best intentions.

- Declare your hopes and intentions, your wishes and your dreams for this space. Let everybody have a turn to

express their wishes in whatever way they choose. Speak
them aloud or whisper them. Recite them or sing them.
Make up a new song or poem. Drum them up. Read on
for a beautiful collection of global blessing prayers and
chants for reference and inspiration.

- Light a candle to ignite and activate your vision, and to
  attract all the good fortune you desire. Again, let each
  person light their own candle.

- Place crystals in the corners of rooms and on shelves,
  windowsills, or mantles to attract your desires and focus
  your blessings. When you lavish your home with love, it
  becomes a gracious receptacle of your dreams, imbued
  with warmth, harmony, health, prosperity, and joy.

STAGE 3.   MAINTAINING THE ENERGY

Now that the energy is cleansed and blessed, it is important
to keep it that way. Here are some ways to absorb any
residual negative energy or any that might accumulate as
time goes by.

- Wet a Blue Ball (this is laundry bluing compressed into
  little balls) with water. Doing so turns it into a washable
  watercolor paint. Draw it along the threshold of all of
  your exterior doorways. In doing so, you are enforcing
  your boundaries and creating a protective barrier against

unwanted energies entering your space, "drawing the line," as it were. Or you can drop a rose of Jericho (also known as a resurrection plant) into a glass or bowl of water and place it at a window or any other spot that seems vulnerable to you. It will absorb any negativity in the area. Periodically flush the water and start again after the rose of Jericho has dried out and closed up again, to keep the space energetically clean.

- Designate a tabletop, shelf, or mantle in your space to serve as an altar, which will be an ever-present reminder of all that you hope for your home and a focal point for your ongoing blessings. Refer to Chapter 6 for some helpful ideas about creating altars.

- Light a candle on your altar to consecrate your new space. The flame will activate your intentions and attract all the good fortune that you desire. A green candle traditionally represents growth, abundance, health, and good luck. A pink one brings in the warmth of loving kindness and comfort and compassionate support. White represents the purity of your intentions and a blank-slate new beginning. Red is for purpose, passion, power, and protection. Use whatever color is meaningful to you and represents your hopes and wishes.

- Have each member of the household add offerings
  of tobacco or rice or corn or pennies or flower petals
  or chocolates or any other items that are symbolic
  of appreciation and thanksgiving. This will serve as a
  constant reminder to maintain an attitude of gratitude
  and keep your own inner energy pure and positive.

- Give each person in the household, as well as each visitor,
  a small pebble or shell or crystal to hold, and ask them to
  make a wish for you and your home. Place these amulets
  on the altar. In this way, you are always connected to the
  love and support of those relationships that you cherish.

- You can put a rose of Jericho in a small bowl of water on your
  altar as well. This is a desert plant that is closed in on itself in
  a tight, dry, fistlike ball when it is in its dormant stage. Once it
  is in the water, it will gradually open to reveal a bright green
  interior that takes in any foul energy. Then when the water
  evaporates, the ball closes in again, digesting the negativity.
  This is a perpetual plant that will open and close for many
  years, keeping your space energized and free of negativity.

- As time goes by, enhance your altar with special personal
  items that you feel are filled with good spirit. These can
  be family photographs, religious images, lucky coins,
  souvenirs, family keepsakes, and/or inspirational quotes. In

this way your altar becomes a living museum of the loving memories that you are creating as you live in your home.

VARIATIONS ON A THEME

The list of ways to personalize your blessings is endless. Feel free to express your intentions in any way that pleases you. Experiment, improvise, ad lib, play!

- Give some thought to how you feel now that you have accomplished a House Blessing of your own design and process. Did it express your intentions? Reflect your sensibilities? How does your home feel to you now? Is there anything you would do differently next time? Are you confident that you will be able to create future Blessings when you feel that they are called for?

See Chapter 9 for a detailed list of ingredients and supplies and how and when to use them in your Blessing ceremony—perhaps there are ingredients you didn't use for the first go-round that you would like to experiment with next time.

BLESSINGS ABOUND

"Blessing" means to infuse something with holiness. Here are some Blessings for the home from cultures around the

world to incorporate into your personalized ceremony.
Feel free to use them if they speak to you. Repeat them
as they are, or change them in a way that expresses your
sentiments. Or let them inspire you to compose a Blessing
of your own that articulates more precisely your desires and
intentions for your space. Your Blessings can be composed
in advance like these, or they can be spontaneous, letting
the energy of the space lead you to convey your hopes and
dreams as you feel them in the moment.

> May the clouds of the Blessed One's spiritual powers,
> His unrivalled knowledge and boundless compassion,
> Pour down upon your house like a monsoon rain,
> Nurturing the roots of your wholesome qualities.
> —Buddhist, Ven. Bhikkhu Bodhi

> May the warm winds of heaven blow softly upon this lens
> (house). May the Great Spirit bless all who enter here.
> —Cherokee

> God, protect our going out and our coming in;
> Let us share the hospitality of this home with all who visit us,
> that those who enter here may know your love and peace.
> —Catholic

We believe in living deeply, laughing often and loving always.
We believe we were brought together to support and care for each
other. We believe in celebrating together—our faith, our heritage,
our traditions. We believe that everyone's feelings count, and that
the uniqueness of each of us strengthens all of us. We believe in
the power of forgiveness to heal and the power of love to carry us
through. We believe in one another, in this family, in this home.

—Author Unknown

May you always be blessed; with walls for the wind,
a roof for the rain, a warm cup of tea by the fire,
laughter to cheer you, those you love near you
and all that your heart might desire.

—Gaelic

May the blessing of God crown this house
where our children go in and out. When they and we go out
and in, let Thou us blessed be.

—German

Facing you, O House, who are facing me, I approach you
peacefully: sacred Fire and Water are within, the main
doors to Cosmic Order.

—Hindu, *Atharva Veda IX, 3*

And Allah has made for you in your homes an abode ...
May the peace and blessings of Allah
be upon us in this house.
—Islamic, *al-Nahl 16:80*

Let no sadness come through this gate,
Let no trouble come to this dwelling,
Let no fear come through this door,
Let no conflict be in this place,
Let this home be filled with the blessing of joy,
and peace.
—Jewish

May this be a good place for us to live again, may it be
happy in this home; may our lives be long and happy in this
home.May I live in this home happily and peacefully and
with respect. May I have a happy life in this hogan. Myself,
my wife, my children, my relatives, whomever may come
into this hogan, may they relax peacefully and rest up. May
all of us have no sickness, no misfortunes.
—Navajo

Bless this house and the souls who go in and out.
—Pennsylvania German

Lord, we ask you to bless this family
with a warm place by the fire when the world is cold,
a light in the window when the way is dark,
a welcoming smile when the road is long,
a haven of love when the day is done.
For the blessing of this home we give thanks.

—Polish

Dwell in peace in the home of your own being, and the
Messenger of Death will not be able to touch you.

—Sikh, Guru Nanak

The Christ presence
Dwelling in this home
and abiding in the heart
Of each one here, is protection
Against disease, accident,
In harmony, or want. Divine Love
Permeates this home. Bringing
Peace, joy, safety, and prosperity.
This home is a haven of peace
And contentment.
Only good abides here.

—Unity

I pray to heaven to bestow the best of blessings on this
house and on all that shall hereafter inhabit it. May none
but honest and wise men ever rule under this roof.
—White House Blessing by President John Adams
*(Franklin D. Roosevelt was so taken with the prayer that he
had it inscribed in the mantel of the East Room fireplace.)*

Touch the lintel and touch the wall,
Nothing but blessings here befall!
Bless the candle that stands by itself,
Bless the book on the mantle shelf,
Bless the pillow for the tired head,
Bless the hearth and the light shed.
Friends who tarry here, let them know
A threefold blessing before they go.
Sleep for weariness—peace for sorrow
Faith in yesterday and tomorrow.
Lintel and windows, sill and wall,
Nothing but good, this place befall.
—Wiccan

It takes hands to build a house,
but only hearts can build a home.
—Author Unknown

This is your home.
Bless it and it will bless you.

I want to remind myself and others that our homes can become sacred places filled with life and meaning. We do not need cathedrals to remind ourselves to experience the sacred.

—Gunilla Norris, *Inviting Silence*

CHAPTER 6

Home Is Where the Heart Is

CREATING SACRED SPACE

Now that your new house has been cleansed and blessed, it is time to think about actually living your life in it and making it your own. This is the fun part!

By putting your personal touch on your room, your apartment, your house, you are claiming it as your domain.

When I was a sophomore in college I had the opportunity to move to New York City with a recent graduate who was going there for a job. The perfect opportunity to fulfill my lifelong dream of living in the Big Apple. We found a typically tiny one-bedroom

Manhattan apartment. She got the bedroom, because she had the job. The living room was mine. A big empty space with white walls, not very cozy for a stranger in a strange land. But I didn't want or need much. A foam mattress on the floor covered with a fabulous black-and-white zebra velour thrift find was both bed and couch. Everything I owned was in a black metal footlocker trunk, which I placed in front of my seat to use as dining table, desk, and altar. I hung a big Yin Yang poster on the wall across from the rest of my "furniture." The final touch was a yellow light bulb plugged directly into the socket near the floor, which cast a warm embrace of a glow. Voila! The room was still not cozy, but that blank-slate decor perfectly matched my state of mind at the time. It was a spare, yet intimate temple for this apprentice-initiate seeking my way in the world. Precisely what I needed for reflection, inspiration, and courage.

Whether we are fully conscious of it or not,
we actually derive countenance and sustenance
from the "atmosphere" of the things we live in or with.
—Frank Lloyd Wright

When you create a living environment that suits your needs and desires, your intentions, your values, and your aesthetics, it will transform your residence into your true home—a sacred space that feeds and focuses your sense of connection, ease, and spiritual support. Such a soulful haven is described as *gemutlich* in German, meaning "cozy, comfortable, pleasant, friendly." *Gemutlich* derives from *gemüt*, which refers to nature, mind, and soul. *Hygge* (pronounced hue-guh) is a Danish word to identify a palpable quality of comfort, coziness, conviviality, contentment, and charm that promotes feelings of well-being. This concept derives from a sixteenth-century Norwegian term, meaning "to comfort" or "to console," and is related to the English word "hug." The warm hug of a *hygge* home is essential in the frozen dark stretches of Nordic winters. And the cheerful embrace of a *hygge* home is equally necessary in the stressful rush and push of urban life.

From the earliest domestic abode, whether a cave, a tent, a lean-to, or an edifice constructed of mud, stones, reeds, branches, hides, or ice, the center of the home has always been the glowing hearth. This fiery place provided warmth from the elements, protection from hungry animals, satisfying cooked food, and a cheerful gathering space. The hearth is the heart of a home. It is the high altar of the art and craft of living well. Its central heat fuels the most basic and profound daily rituals of nurturance, sustenance, support, and communion. The hearth stokes the healthy spirit that comes from physical ease and emotional fulfillment. The holy hearth nourishes the human heart. Like the hearth, our heart is our central fire, the pulsing forge of our most authentic self. It is the furnace from which radiates the heat, the power, and the passion of our lives, and the warmth of our being.

The kitchen is still the energetic center of any soulful home. No matter how large, well designed, and sumptuously decorated the other rooms of a house might be, it is the kitchen where people inevitably want to gather and spend time, whether cooking, eating, popping a beer, doing homework, finger painting, paying bills, or playing cards. At even the most luxurious cocktail parties, people are drawn, one by one, into the kitchen until the entire festivity has migrated there—folks hanging out, perched on the counters, leaning against the sink, pouring their drinks directly from the fridge, lighting their smokes from the stove burner, making themselves completely at home.

My fondest childhood Thanksgiving memory involves what transpired after the fancy dinner—which was served on the good china at the dining room table, covered in damask and graced with candles, flowers, and cloth napkins—was finished. The women and girls, mother, grandmother, aunt, and cousins, cleared the table and repaired to the kitchen to clean up, after which we always ended up sitting around the Formica kitchen table, picking shreds of turkey with our fingers off of the carcass that had been removed from the serving platter and returned to the roasting pan. Happy as pigs in mud, we stayed there snacking and chatting for hours.

Home is not just a place where you go to sleep, it is a primary part of your life and has a vital effect on how you live it. Your abode is the headquarters where you plan and stage your life. Your home defines and describes you. It directs your attention. The surest way to create a friendly, supportive ambience, one that feels as good as it looks, is to use only furnishings and objects that you truly need and really love.

Surround yourself with colors, textures, and meaningful objects that soothe, inspire, excite, and delight you. When you have established such an agreeable place for yourself, you will be rewarded by the simple satisfying sensual pleasure of just being there. The beauty and comfort that you experience will imbue this, your most intimate environment, with a palpable sense of contentment that mirrors and magnifies your own.

Your home will also reflect any change in the circumstances of your life and will need to be adapted to accommodate them. Creating a new or renovated living environment is a perfect metaphor for redirecting the focus of your life. A newly divorced client contacted me a while ago for advice as to how she could make her house more cozy and nicer to be in now that she is living there alone, a very common situation. She said she had cleansed the space, but now she felt as though she was "living in an empty theater." Starting with an empty theater is a great metaphor for redesigning a way of life. Your home is the proscenium on which you can stage and star in the production of your own life. My advice for her, and anyone else whose living situations are in flux, is not to feel that you have to redecorate it all at once. Your home will change as you do and will fill little by little when your life has filled out again. By simply living in the house, you will possess it and enliven it with your spirit. And once your spirit owns the space, it will speak to you and let you know precisely what you need and what you desire in order to be happy living in the home that is truly yours.

It is tempting to want a complete change done fast right now this minute, because that would mean that you had already transformed yourself and were settled into a new stage in your life, as it were. But be assured that your personal makeover will come to pass from the very process of your homemaking. So, burrow in, make soup, put on music, light some sweet incense, and putter around. Do projects. Live your life and make creative work there. Cook and eat and read and dance and dream there. Relax. You are home. And there is no place like home!

> I think the most significant work we ever do
> in our whole world, in our whole life, is done
> within the four walls of our own home.
> —June Cotner, *House Blessings*

I never could understand how people could design all of the tiniest details of a house on paper and then build precisely from those plans. How can you possibly know what you want and where you want something until after you have inhabited the space? How can you be sure exactly where you want your bathtub, a window seat, a particular drawer or light switch or outlet, until you experience the movement of sun and shadows as well as the family dynamics and your own habits, and requirements show you the way?

ORGANIC CHANGE

Instead, I prefer to shape my home around myself like a nautilus grows her shell around her soft tissue as her body expands. I add to or alter my surroundings very gradually as I find things that I like, that I need, that I make myself. I am a bowerbird or magpie, foraging for the fripperies with which to decorate my nest. And each new thing that I bring inside demands to be set into the living environment with thought, feeling, and intention. This ritual of placement assures that each item, each addition, each replacement, each adjustment, each improvement makes a relevant statement to me. Nothing superfluous, nothing not a reflection of my own taste and experience. As the English designer William Morris counseled, "Have nothing in your home that you do not know to be useful or believe to be beautiful." My home is a living Museum of Who I Am Now At This Particular Time. As my life is lived and changes are made, my living space evolves in response. And so will yours. The new feeling you create in your space will lift your mood and your energy and spirits will soar.

A house is no home unless it contains food and
fire for the mind as well as the body.
—Benjamin Franklin

HOME ALONE

A house or apartment that is home to more than one person is by definition a communal space, an interactive place that encourages the sharing of meals, conversation, affection, and chores. But sometimes, all of the coming and going, the clutter and chatter just become too much, and we long for some uninterrupted privacy, peace, and quiet. That deep spiritual source at the very center of our soul cries out, for the sake of our sanity, to inhabit a special, sanctified space of our own creation to use for our own purposes, "a room of our own," as Virginia Woolf put it. This is our go-to safe space, our *querencia*, our hermit cave, our sanctuary for repose and renewal, a private, personal space where we can be happily at home with ourselves doing whatever it is we want to do there. The personal space you crave might be a meditation room, library, office, or sewing room; a yoga, dance, art, or music studio; a playroom; a workshop; a man cave; or a she-shed. The possibilities are endless.

Ideally, each member of the family can have their own private place within the collective household. This doesn't mean that each person gets to have an entire room for their personal use, unless your home can accommodate that. If there is no space for an entire room of your own, nor enough money to do a major renovation of your space, improvise. You can create a private area in many creative, inexpensive ways. Children are genius when it comes to doing just that. Kids build forts, clubhouses, playhouses, and dollhouses out of whatever is at hand. Take some rope and a blanket and you've got a tent, pad the closet floor with pillows for a comfy hideaway. Crawl under the stairs or the porch or the bed and enter the hidden cavern. A private space might also mean that each person is guaranteed a certain amount of time alone in a shared room. Or you might install a curtain between the twin beds of a room that siblings share as a simple solution. Or create a private-time corner in the living room or den or porch with curtains or screens and pillows inside. A perfect hidden space for taking a nap or reading or just daydreaming. An enforced quiet hour every day without music or media or talking can accomplish the same sense of freedom and privacy to be alone with a book, a project, a meditation, or your own thoughts.

When I was in junior high school, I commandeered the attic, where no one ever went, and established my secret chapel, which I decorated with handwritten affirmations, though I didn't then know the word for these penned and drawn blessings. My cherished hideaway was furnished with a desk made from an upturned wooden box, on which sat my mother's big old black secretary typewriter, and a cushion on the floor to sit on. I spent long hours over several years enjoying my secret Self-sessions up there, lost in thought, writing in my diary, composing poems, and pondering life's big questions.

I still create tiny enclosed room environments inside my huge flexible loft space to house a particular project I am working on. Before I began writing *The Queen of My Self*, I carved out a minuscule six-foot-square space in a corner of my studio using shoji screens. I jury-rigged a desk arrangement and a place for my files and books. The screens are covered with my collection of fabulous 1940s bark cloth that I had been saving for years in order to use for something really special. This would be it! The Queen's Chambers, I called it. Inside was my sovereignty altar filled with inspirational images, amulets, totems, and tokens of majestic feminine power. I suppose spending so much time and energy constructing a writing room could be mistaken for procrastination, a detour away from actually writing. But creating that royal retreat throne room was instrumental in informing and inspiring my writing about the Queen Archetype. It was probably the most important part of the process of that several-year project. The concepts, the writing, the spirit flowed freely from the regal feeling that my little room encouraged in me.

As you spend time in your new digs, you will find your favorite corners and discover one or more specific spots where, for some mysterious reason, you feel especially good, like you really belong there. Those are your power points where your energy is most focused. There is a place in every space, a particular location in your environment where you feel the most comfortable and at ease. That is your *sitio*, the Spanish word for "space" or "place." *Your* place. Your special place. Your safe spot, your sacred space.

In *The Teachings of Don Juan*, Carlos Casteneda describes how Don Juan, his Yaqui shaman mentor, assigns him the lesson of locating his *sitio*. Don Juan had him get down on the floor of the porch and roll around until he could identify his perfect spot. Once he found his place, he was supposed to spread his bedroll there and spend the night. But after crawling around for a very long time without locating his power place, Carlos felt frustrated and foolish, and eventually just drifted off to sleep. In the morning, Don Juan came out of the house and congratulated him for finding his *sitio*. As it happened, his body and spirit had automatically stopped looking and just relaxed when he was in his proper place.

When thinking about claiming a room of your own that would feel comfortable and supportive, relaxing and inspiring, locating your *sitio* is a good place to start. That vibrant energetic spot is the seat of your personal power and, like the hearth, a source of nurturing energy to fuel your creative and spiritual impulses. Make an effort to identify your *sitio*.

Here are some suggestions to help you on this spiritual treasure hunt:

- Put some meditative music on, dim the lights, and walk, dance, slide, crawl, or roll slowly through your home. You might want to close or squint your eyes so that you can concentrate on what you feel rather than what you see.

- Do you feel yourself drawn to a particular area or corner? How did it attract you? What does it feel like to stand or sit on? You will know when you find it. This is your *sitio*, your own sacred space. This is the place where you can feel most strongly your connections to the energy of the earth, to spirit, and to your inner best Self.

- Claim this space as sacred. Embrace that space. You will want to connect with and acknowledge the good energy that you feel there. Depending on what your intention for the space is, this is where you will put your bed, or your desk, drawing table, easel, dining table, library, or meditation pillow. The good spirit of this spot will energize whatever activity is closest to your heart.

Your *sitio* need not be big. It can be as large as a room; as small as a yoga mat, pillow, rug, or chair; as contained and hidden as a closet. It can be a sitting area or desk space in a larger room. It can be under a dormer in the attic, or outside in the yard or on the porch.

One of my spiritual counseling clients lives in a typically small Manhattan apartment with her husband and eleven-year-old daughter. She does not have any space at all to call her own. She was desperate for a private moment, a quiet time out for some simple contemplation, some concentrated focus on her thoughts. I asked, was there enough room in the bedroom for a chair? There was. And what's more, her brother had serendipitously just sent her a gift certificate for IKEA. So she bought the most comfortable, comforting cushy chair with a high back, which she turns to the corner for privacy as she writes in her journal. Her corner is her sacrosanct refuge surrounded by a moat. Teeming with crocodiles.

ALTARED SENSIBILITY

Every life needs its altar. It may be in a quiet nook,
it may be a moment in the day, or a mood of the heart...
but somewhere the spirit life must have its altar.
From there, life gains its poise and direction.
—Esther B. York in *The Temple in the House*
by Anthony Lawlor

You might want to sanctify your home and your special place within it by creating a personal or family altar and placing it where the energy seems right for it—its *sitio*. Your altar is the energetic heart center of your home, your room, or your *sitio* that pulses with the spirit of your hopes, dreams, and intentions for this space and for all who live and visit there. Your *sitio* altar is your home within your home.

In ancient times the home altar was often placed at the hearth, or heart center, of the home. In this position the energy of the altar is radiated throughout the house. Another traditional place for an altar is near the entrance to a dwelling. Placed here, the altar greets you when you first enter the home, and it is the last thing you see as you leave it to go out into the world. This creates a powerful template for experience. The subconscious mind is programmed continually in this way to recreate the imagery of the altar throughout the day.

Altars are not necessarily religious, but an arrangement of objects and images that are personally meaningful and hold special significance. You probably already have at least one altar, without thinking of it in such terms. Most folks have assemblages of family photos, pictures of friends and pets and vacations, spiritual symbols, inspiring images of nature, keepsakes, souvenirs, and various tokens of sentimental value. Most home altars are displayed on bookcases, tabletops, dressing tables, and desks. It used to be popular to display such an altar on top of the television set—not possible with flat screens today. It is also possible to contain altars in boxes. Think of the cigar box treasure chest that held your childhood relics and objects of veneration.

- Sanctify your home and *sitio* by creating an altar with some special, personally significant items—photographs of loved ones, memorabilia, stones gathered from travels, artwork of your children—whatever you find to be inspiring. The visual display you create will continually remind you of the purpose of your best intentions for your space and your life. The amount of room and privacy you have will determine the size and form of your altar.

- You can construct a formal altar with many holy icons, lucky charms, inspiring images and texts, offerings, and candles, or you can discreetly place certain personally (and privately) precious items on your desktop or dresser top, bookshelf, or windowsill.

- If you share your space at work or in a crowded household, you can create an altar inside of a drawer or cabinet or closet and it will be private and completely hidden to all but you. I keep an altar in an old wooden medicine cabinet, opened for my eyes only.

- Claim and defend adequate blocks of time to spend in your *sitio* or at your altar so that you might engage with your Self on a regular basis. Use your sacred time and space to write in your journal, listen to music, meditate, do your yoga or exercises, dance, read, daydream, or nap.

- With Self-engagement and development on your mind, any time can be auspicious and any place a sanctuary. All you need do is claim it as so.

Some keep the Sabbath going to church
I keep it staying at home,
With a bobolink for a chorister,
And an orchard for a dome.
—Emily Dickinson

One day while walking down Bleecker Street, I came upon a gypsy fortuneteller's storefront and became transfixed by the fantastic arrangement that was meticulously displayed in the window. The energy that it generated was completely compelling. After some time of my standing there staring, she came out to entice me in for a reading. I demurred, telling her, "No thanks. I was just admiring your altar." "My what?" she replied. "Oh, you mean how I fix things." Yes, it was the stunning effect of how she put it all together that was so inspired and powerfully focused.

I love altars. I love seeking them out in museums and places of worship. I especially love creating altars—for every purpose, for every occasion. I have an inspiration and encouragement altar over and around my work desk. I have an ancestor altar in my bedroom and also one dedicated to love. There are altars for healing, for abundance, for personal power, and for Mother Earth reverence in my ritual consulting room. My entire kitchen is an altar to the sacred hearth, the flaming heart of health, home, and hospitality. My guest bathroom is a floor-to-ceiling folk shrine to the compassionate goddess Tonantzin, better known today as the Mexican Our Lady of Guadalupe.

Do you have an altar in your home?
Is it intentional?
Do you recognize any altars that you have created without really thinking about it?
What is sacred to you?
What is healing?
What is inspiring?
What is comforting?
What are your intentions in life?
For what do you feel gratitude?
Are these thoughts and feelings reflected in your altar?

The answers to these questions are the building blocks of your altar. They are what make an altar personal and powerful. There are no rules about setting up an altar. There are no wrong ways—just follow your intuition.

When you listen to your inner voice, your altar will perfectly reflect your deepest, most authentic best Self. And it will continue to be relevant and supportive of your spiritual needs, until which time that it no longer is. When your altar ceases to speak to you and spirit you away to a deep place of internal connection and reverence, it will need updating. Your altar is not set in stone. Change it as you change, like your hairstyle, wardrobe, or decor, so that it can continue to express the spirit of your hopes, dreams, and visions for your space and for all who live and visit there.

KEEPING HOUSE

Now that you have cleared the old energy from your space and replaced it with the spirit generated by your blessings, and now that you have identified your *sitio* and installed an altar to charge the atmosphere, you will certainly want to keep the energy in your home feeling fresh and positive, comforting and uplifting.

Part of housekeeping is keeping the good energy flowing. The artful Hindu system of *Vashtu* is concerned with aligning each element in any space with its proper location, which allows the energy to circulate smoothly. This alignment, where nothing feels out of place or jarring, creates a powerful rhythm that moves easily around each individual object and from room to room. The free flow of energy establishes an aura of dependable predictability, which in turn promotes feelings of security and comfort. The rhythm of the house mirrors the rhythmic cycles of the universe, which are also predictable: the sequence of light and dark, hot and cold, wet and dry; the phases of the moon; and the seasonal changes, the observance of which encourages a spiritual connection of your home with the natural world.

You can draw on feng shui principles to govern the spatial orientation and arrangement of your objects in relation to the flow of energy, or chi, with the goal of creating balance with the spiritual forces of the natural world. This art of harmonious placement offers some basic suggestions for creating a well-balanced, peaceful environment:

- Clear your clutter. Disorder in your surroundings saps time and energy and blocks clear thinking. It also prevents an easy flow of energy.

- Invite as much light and air inside as you can. The air clears a foggy mental atmosphere and the light simply lightens your spirit. Add plants to purify the air and inspire connection to the universal life force.

- Enter and leave your house by the front door. This is how the chi, the energy, enters. By using a back door or the garage, you limit how much good and bountiful energy can come inside.

- Oil your squeaks, especially those on the front door. If the door sounds like it is crying, it will scare the good chi away.

- Keep the bathroom door closed and the seat down, lest your good fortune be flushed away.

- Put your bed in what feng shui calls "the commanding position." That is, facing the door, but not directly in line with it. This serves as protection during the long hours when you are asleep.

- Clean your windows. If the front door is the mouth of the house, the windows are the eyes, and they need to be clean so you can be clear sighted.

- Cover the TV in the bedroom when you are not watching it. Even when it is not on, it emits low-energy X-ray radiation and electromagnetic field rays into your home that are energetically disruptive.

SPICK AND SPAN

Cleaning is the process of removing dirt from any space, surface, object, or subject, thereby exposing beauty, potential, truth, and sacredness.
—Tolulope Ilesanmi, Owner of Zenith Cleaners, Montreal, Canada

I grew up in the 1950s, the era of supposedly happy homemakers like June Cleaver who donned a shirtwaist dress, pearls, and pumps and made sure the seams of her stockings were straight before starting to vacuum. Until the relatively recent influence of feminist thought, housecleaning was deemed to be solely the responsibility of women, and thus undervalued and generally demeaned. Cleaners, whether members of the domestic family or corporate employees, are relatively invisible. Yet they perform tasks that are crucial for our spiritual as well as physical well-being and comfort. Though considered to be menial labor, cleaning has an almost alchemical effect of making and remaking a home or any space anew, magically transforming it with focused care through consistent tidying, dusting, mopping, waxing, cleaning, polishing.

Clearing and cleaning your personal space can result in enhanced mental clarity and an improved memory. By cleaning your home, you honor it. Cleaning is a loving, caring practice that makes a big difference. When you clean, you heal, restore, renew, transform, and beautify your most favorite possessions and intimate surroundings. In doing so, you cleanse, restore, and transform yourself in both tangible and intangible ways. Cleaning can be a sacred practice if you allow yourself to be fully present in the process. As the Buddhists say, "Chop wood, carry water." Do what you are doing while you are doing it. Concentrate. "Be here now," counsels Ram Dass. Pay reverent attention to the metaphoric intention of your task. As Tolulope Ilesanmi reminds us, "When we mop a floor, wipe a counter top, scrub a toilet, dust a table, it is not so much about the physical dirt we are removing from the object, surface, or space. It is about the dirt we are removing within us." If your home is your sanctuary, taking care of it by cleaning is a form of prayer.

Despite the fact that I loathe vacuuming, I am a happy homemaker and inveterate altarista. I love my home. I love my altars and I actually love to clean them. One of my greatest pleasures is to turn up some jivey hypnotic music and go at it. Not a thorough cleaning every day, mind you, but some bit of ordering, arranging, freshening, some loving attention and appreciation to my precious temple. The best housekeeping tip I ever received was from an old colleague and mentor. She was a famous choreographer and traveled far and wide to work. She also raised three daughters in a huge homey loft that always looked perfectly organized and sparkling clean. She said that she never did more than forty-five minutes of housework a day. With that minimal amount of concerted effort you can accomplish quite a bit, so things remain orderly and you never have to do an exhausting marathon cleaning day.

While I was working on this chapter, it occurred to me with crashing awareness and shame that here I was devoting the greater part of my attention to writing about creating and maintaining a sacred space, while I was neglecting my own. My house was a mess. What a disturbing paradox. Then suddenly one afternoon when I was deep in a paragraph, I was brought back to my senses by a deafening explosion in the kitchen. What the . . . ? Nothing seemed wrong until I opened the fridge to a shocking sight. Somehow a heavy unopened jar had slid off the top shelf and had fallen onto the glass shelf below, shattering it. There was glass everywhere, shards in the drawers, in the food, on the floor. It was totally unnerving, way too much to deal with. I closed the door and went to bed.

I was calmer in the morning and swept the floor and struggled with the refrigerator shelves and drawers until I finally figured out how to remove them. I tossed the food, emptied the shelves, got rid of the glass, and put it all back together again. As I was washing each jar and bottle before returning it to its place, I realized that I was smiling. It felt wonderful to be domestic again and care for my surroundings and belongings. While thinking and writing gives me great joy, I was reminded of this other, more intimate kind of bliss. Ever since that jarring realization, I take a break from the book every hour or so to do some homey task—wash the dishes, water the plants, put a load in the washer, dust my altars—a most satisfying arrangement that adds reciprocal depth and resonance to both occupations. These slipped-in bits of focused care and domestic maintenance are not onerous tasks, but rather intentional acts of love that honor the sanctity of my home.

- What cleaning rituals do you practice?

- What cleaning rituals do you enjoy?

- Do you take pleasure in caring for your home?

- What are your favorite home-keeping actions?

I always wondered why the makers leave housekeeping and cooking out of their tales. Isn't it what all the great wars and battles are fought for—so that at day's end a family may eat together in a peaceful house?

—Ursula K. Le Guin

This is your home.
Honor its sanctity.

Home is a notion that only nations of the homeless
fully appreciate and only the uprooted
comprehend.

—Wallace Stegner, *Angle of Repose*

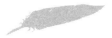

CHAPTER 7

Out of House and Home

We identify with our home in a very profound way. This is why, for most people, moving is one of life's most emotionally loaded and disruptive experiences, provoking a deep-seated dread of being uprooted, of not belonging. The poet Sylvia Plath described that scary feeling this way: "the danger is that in this move toward new horizons and far directions that I may lose what I have now, and not find anything except loneliness." Changing our residence elicits a resistance against forfeiting the known, and accentuates the fear of the unknown. Leaving home voluntarily is hard enough. But when people lose their homes due to death, divorce, financial reversal, urban gentrification, fire, or natural disaster, the pain of being dislocated, displaced is overwhelming. The ground under their feet is less solid, their protective citadel no longer secure. Their sense of Self is decimated. I know that feeling.

PARADISE LOST

When I was twenty-two and living alone for the first time, my tenement storefront loft burst into flames while I was taking a nap. Luckily, I lived on the ground floor and made it out, barefoot in my pajamas, physically unharmed. But I lost everything that I owned, along with one of my cats. For months afterward, I lived in a discombobulated daze, somehow able to muddle through my job without sobbing, barely getting by. I was so disconnected that for months every time I looked into a mirror I saw a complete stranger. I literally did not recognize myself. Who is that? Who am I? Who am I now? It was as though I had left my soul in the burning building and was walking around without it, unfocused and aimless, rootless and homeless. In such dire circumstances it is easy to forget who you are and where you belong.

Yet, I was lucky. I happened to live right across the street from The Catholic Worker charity, which immediately gave me a sweater, a pair of jeans, and some sneakers. The Red Cross arrived right after the Fire Department and found me a temporary room with two months' free lodging in a welfare hotel, so I had a place to sleep that very night. And I had a job, which meant I could save money for a security deposit and first month's rent of a really horrible furnished apartment. It was tiny and ugly, but it was mine for a time. I had the key. It was home for now. I finally had some personal space and a certain stability that had been stolen by the fire. There, I could finally grieve for my losses, thank my lucky stars, pick up the pieces of my broken confidence, and get myself together to begin again.

But what about the nearly three quarters of a million folks in the United States today with nowhere to call home and no prospects for having one? My own unsettling situation made me sensitive to the plight of the truly homeless. Someone recently said to me, "When you are homeless, you don't have a key. When you don't have a key, you are not a person." Our culture equates a key with autonomy, adulthood, and ownership. If you don't have a key, by this rubric you are clearly not an autonomous adult who owns things. You are thus without status, a non-person in society's eyes. A derelict, a tramp, a bum. A nobody.

Being homeless means you have no place to live, nor roof over your head, and certainly no door. Roofless, you are exposed, vulnerable to the elements and to predators, yet invisible to passersby who avert their gaze. When you are roofless, you are rootless. Without a door you have no privacy, no autonomy, and no protection. Being doorless means you are also keyless. Without a key you couldn't lock the door even if you had one. When a child draws a picture of a house without a door, it is considered by psychologists to indicate insecurity. By contrast, a drawing of a house with a door and a doorknob suggests a trusting openness. Without a door you can't close the world out, nor can you invite it in. Doorless, you can't open your space in friendly welcome like any other humane being can. Ironically, not having a door is more isolating than having one.

Doors are a wonderful invention
second to the wheel! Open one
at certain times and you will let fresh air in,
a guest as sweet as Spring, which has been
walking among flowers or marshes. If a gush
of Winter comes, you can—in a rush—

close it quickly with a fervent bang!
You'll like doors—once you get the hang
of how they work! They have the terrific clout
to give two different worlds—In and Out—
to you, at will. The trick, now and again,
is knowing what to do with them—and when!
—Helen Harrington, *Whimsy on Doors*

When a series of explosions in April of 1986 destroyed the nuclear reactor at the power station in Chernobyl in the Ukraine, Soviet Socialist Republic, the population was forced by armed soldiers to evacuate. They were forbidden to take anything with them, because every object was hot from radiation, a ticking nuclear bomb way too dangerous to handle. But despite the restrictions, which were for their own safety and for the safety of anyone else they would encounter from now on, folks secreted heirlooms, photos, and homegrown food on their person to take with them in a desperate attempt to maintain some connection to their homes and villages. What would you take if you had to run?

One of the most poignant passages in the extraordinary book *Voices From Chernobyl: The Oral History of a Natural*

Disaster, by Svetlana Alexievich, tells of one Chernobyl resident lugging the door of his house on his back as he left. His door was his most treasured possession. Each of his childhood years, along with those of his siblings and his own children, was marked in chalk on that door. And when his father died, they unhinged the door and laid him out on it until his coffin was ready, as was the custom in his village. He referred to the door of his home as his holy talisman. It had been the gateway to all that was precious in his life, both inside and outside of his house. It was unthinkable to leave it behind. Without it, he would be doorless.

On a list of top stressful life situations, moving house comes in third place, after death of a spouse and divorce, but way more stressful than dealing with a major illness, loss of a job, or financial setback. If losing a home is such a devastating experience, losing a homeland is ever more excruciating. How many millions of people have we watched on television over the years as they flee for their lives from the ravages of tornadoes, hurricanes, earthquakes, droughts, famines, floods, terror, and war? The horrifying scene is all too familiar: Throngs of refugees with just the clothes on their backs, maybe a few things in their pockets, panic in their eyes, and broken hearts, leaving everything they had ever known and running toward…what? Where? When? How? There are entire generations of people in unstable nations all over the world who live their whole lives without ever having had a home. A Palestinian college friend of mine was born in a refugee camp, and half a century later his family is still there, unable to leave with nowhere to go.

Thirty years after my fire and brief sample of being homeless, I was exposed to another mini refugee experience. On September 11, 2001, my honey and I were staying in a charming cluster of cabins on the shore of the upper St. Lawrence River in Quebec on our way to the Gaspé. It was out of season and we were the only guests. It was a beautiful blue-sky sunny day, we were on vacation, and the river was alive with whales. What could be more idyllic? We decided to stay another day and went to the office to pay. The television was on and broadcasting an endless loop of jetliners flying into the World Trade Center. What? Here we were in a tranquil paradise; how could we comprehend the horrors we were watching with tear-blurred eyes? Not only was my country, my city, attacked, the World Trade Center Plaza had been my public altar, the site of fifteen years of my equinox and solstice ceremonies, now completely obliterated. For me, this was intensely, painfully personal.

What happened to the people I worked with there? The directors who sponsored my events, and their staff? The custodial team who helped me set up and clean up? Did they make it through alive?

Of course our first thought was to get home. Immediately. But there was no way home. The borders were sealed. Planes were grounded. No trains. No cars to rent, and worse, no contact. The phone lines were dead and this remote village had no Wi-Fi. We spent an entire week in the parking lot of the gas station that had the only payphone, trying to call home, but we were never able to get through. We had no idea of what was happening in the days after the eleventh of September. We were stuck where we were with only a tourist vocabulary guide and my eleventh-grade French lessons trying to translate the heavily accented Québécois enough to understand the news. We were desperate for connection. What is it like back home? In the city? At my loft? How is my precious dog? My bird? My plants? My friends? As we watched the footage of thousands of people running across the Brooklyn Bridge to safety, I couldn't help but think of all the televised images of refugees that I had seen over the decades—millions upon millions of refugees and displaced people fleeing their homes, their villages, their cities, on their heartbreaking passage through hell, toward prayed-for safety, a roof, an open door, a welcome mat.

> Give me your tired, your poor,
> Your huddled masses yearning to breathe free,
> The wretched refuse of your teeming shore.
> Send these, the homeless, tempest-tost to me,
> I lift my lamp beside the golden door!
> —Emma Lazarus, *The New Colossus*,
> enshrined at the base of the Statue of Liberty

I identified with their emotional plight. We, too, were exiled in limbo, fraught with fear, separated from everything familiar, a different kind of prisoner in a different kind of war. We couldn't go home, either. But thankfully, our experience, though terrifying, was short lived. And unlike the many millions of refugees and displaced people forced to abandon their homes and their homelands who are, at any given moment, on the move or in camps around the world, we were in safe and comfortable surroundings, complete with a roof, a door, and a key. We had clean clothes, credit cards, and passports. We also had an endless supply of French café and stellar *pain au chocolat* to keep us going. We were very, very lucky. After a week, we were finally able to catch a train back to New York. But I couldn't stop thinking about being stranded in an unfamiliar place, not able to speak the language, with only the belongings in my bag, while my city, my homeland was burning, and with no way to go home—not even a way of knowing whether home was still there and if my friends and neighbors, my animals and my computer with thirty years of work on it, were safe. What if none of it survived? What if there was nothing to return to?

> I washed the house. Bleached the stones.
> You need to leave some bread on the table
> and some salt, in a little plate, and three spoons,
> as many spoons as there are souls in the house.
> All so we could come back.
> —Chernobyl Refugee

MOTHERLAND

Shekhinah is the feminine face of the divine presence in Judaism, a Mother Goddess, if you will. Her name means "domicile." The Semitic root meaning is "to settle, inhabit, or dwell" and is used frequently to refer to birds' nesting and nests, and can also refer to "neighbor." The Hebrew word *mishkan*, meaning "tabernacle," is a derivative of the same root and is used in the sense of a dwelling-place that creates a sacred proximity to the *Shekhinah* and an enhanced sense of God.

Home is more than a specific dwelling. It is also the land itself, as well as the people who populate it and the culture it inspires. Homeland is our origin, our identity, our ethos, our stories, our nostalgia. The sentiment inspired by the term, the concept, of Motherland evokes primal memories of our first home, the womb. Motherland represents all the nurturing aspects of home: warmth, protection, belonging, acceptance, affection, caring. Motherland is where we were born, the land of our forebearers, the Motherly Earth Herself, who nourishes our bodies and our spirits with food and fodder grown in the fertile soil made rich with the bones of our ancestors and the buried placentas of our children. These mother roots are as strong as umbilical cords that connect the lineage of generations to each other and to their mutual birthplace.

I once bought a way-too-big bag of potatoes, which I knew I could never eat before they spoiled, so I brought some to a neighbor. Her visiting mother answered the door and when she took the potatoes in her hands, she smelled them and then licked her fingers. She told me they were from the county in Alabama where she was born. She knew by the smell and the taste of the dirt. When I got home I checked the potato bag and sure enough, they were!

Home is also the Mother Earth womb tomb that will one day cradle our bodies in death. The concepts of death and of home have been widely connected for millennia. For Christians, death is going home to God in Heaven. A Homegoing is a traditional Christian African American funeral celebration that originated in the time of slavery, when the displaced, shackled Africans believed that they would return to their ancestral homeland across the great water when they die. Sojourner Truth jubilantly declared, "I am not going to die, I'm going home like a shooting star." Tecumseh, an eighteenth-century Shawnee warrior and chief, proclaimed, "Sing your death song and die like a hero going home." "Maybe death, when it comes, is simply another longing for home," wrote British novelist Anita Brookner.

When we contemplate our own death most people imagine dying at home, in our own bed, cosseted and embraced by loved ones. Very often, hospitalized critically ill end-stage patients choose to go home, where they feel they belong, to die in peace and dignity. Even though my dying mother was already at home and in her bed, in her last days, she would whisper with longing, "Home. I want to go home."

We are all visitors to this time, this place. We are just passing through. Our purpose here is to observe, to learn, to grow, to love...and then we return home.
—Australian Aboriginal Proverb

This emotional life-and-death connection with the Motherland, with Mother Earth, is shared widely across cultures. The Inuit people, who live around the Arctic Circle, have long resisted misguided attempts by the governments of Canada, Greenland, Russian Lapland, Siberia, and the United States to relocate these nomadic hunters to permanent settlements. These resettlement efforts have not always been successful, as the displaced people languish when they are separated from their sacred *nunatuarigapku*, or homeland, alive as it is with ancestral spirits. Anthropologists tell of hunters abandoning their newly built quarters in towns and villages to return to live in their abandoned camps.

When you live outside your village, you leave your soul.
You can't take me from my mother;
you can't take me from my motherland.
Motherland is Motherland.
—Chernobyl Refugee

After sixty years of living and voting in the United States after having escaped rampaging Cossacks, my gramma still attended meetings of what she called the "Mizricher Society," folks who had also lived in the Międzyrzec area in what is now Poland. She identified with them, although she did not really know these people and had absolutely nothing in common with them, except that they were her *Landsmanns*, from the old country, still connected by an ancient memory of a mutual motherland and a way of life lost. This condition is called *hiraeth* (n.) in Welsh: it means "homesickness for a home to which you cannot return, a home which maybe never was; the nostalgia, the yearning, the grief for the lost places of your past."

An evacuee from Hurricane Katrina in New Orleans, where she had moved from Pennsylvania, said about returning to Philadelphia after having lost everything to the storm, "Coming home to family and friends was a blessing. When I left I just wanted to get away from Philadelphia. When I came back I was just happy to be able to come home. So many people had nowhere to go." When Miriam Makeba, the fabulous singer and human rights worker, was finally allowed to return to South Africa after having lived in exile in the United States, she said, "In the mind, in the heart, I was always home. I always imagined, really, going back home."

> We are all strangers in a strange land, *longing for home*,
> but not quite knowing what or where home is. ...
> is a strange, sweet familiarity that vanishes
> almost as soon as it *comes*...
> —Madeleine L'Engle

Not ever being able to return home is unbearable. Much of Chernobyl had died and been buried—people, animals, crops, whole houses, trees, and the contaminated soil itself had been interred deep underground in the Motherland. But despite the danger and against all common sense, some Chernobyl refugees, older women mostly, chose to return to their villages and, they hoped, their own homes. They evaded armed guards, snuck back to their doomed land, their poisoned forests, their incinerated gardens, their own small plots of dirt that had always sustained them, and where they hoped to lie for eternity when they die. They moved right back in as if nothing had happened. One woman expressed it this way: "Even if it's poisoned by radiation, it's still my home. There's no place else they need us. Even a bird loves its nest."

"The Babushkas," as they are known, who returned to their ancestral homes in the zone of radiation, are thriving in their beloved Motherland. The women live as they always have. They grow and eat potatoes, onions, beets, cabbage. Their crops root them to the earth. They keep a few chickens, a goat, and maybe a cow. They forage for mushrooms and berries. And though everything they eat or touch is irradiated, they are not dying of cancer, but simply of old age, a stroke, a heart attack. They are hale and hearty, happy at home, where they belong. These old wives have been living about a decade longer than those Chernobylites who were relocated and living in exile and so-called safety.

Uprooted plants sometimes die rather than thrive when they are transplanted. People are no different. Anita Shreve writes in *The Weight of Water*, "I remain quite certain that souls, which take root in a particular geography, cannot be successfully transplanted. I believe that these roots, these tiny fibrous filaments, will almost inevitably dry and wither in the new soil, or send the plant into sudden and irretrievable shock."

Relocation doesn't work out so well if your roots have been severed. Many of the refugees who stayed away from Chernobyl after the accident were resettled in faraway villages and towns that were not and never would be home, and where they feel they don't belong. The flip side of belonging is not belonging. Such intense bonding and identification can be exclusionary if you are a stranger or different in some way. This insular divide can grow to become xenophobic, racist, sexist, and anti anyone who is not like you. The folks displaced by Chernobyl were forced to live among strangers who had strange ways. They could not assimilate, nor did they want to. As a result they suffer from long-term anxiety, depression, and disrupted social networks, the same PTSD traumas experienced by displaced people everywhere. They are homesick and heartsick, which has deleterious effects on the health of the body. These are the ones who are dying of radiation-induced cancers. This is not surprising. Many studies have shown the strong link between happiness and longevity. The opposite is also true. Depression and pessimism kill.

Sometimes I feel like a motherless child
Sometimes I feel like a motherless child
Sometimes I feel like a motherless child
A long way from home, a long way from home
—Traditional Negro Spiritual

PARADISE FOUND

In recent years, Chernobyl has been repopulated with hundreds of thousands of refugees, who have fled from wars and political turmoil in Chechnya, Tajikistan, Georgia, and Azerbaijan, seeking sanctuary and tranquility in the abandoned fields and peaceful pastures surrounding Chernobyl. It seemed an Eden for sore souls. There were some surviving empty homes, still sturdy, to shelter their families. The forest was alive with (diseased) birds and beasts to hunt and (poisonous) mushrooms, plants, and berries to pick. The gardens could be brought back to life, and so could their spirits, now that they were far from so much unrelenting terror and violence. "I prefer living with radiation over living in a war zone," said one former resident of Chernobyl.

Many years ago, I opened my life and my Healing Haven home to a ten-year-old foster son, a frightened and angry fugitive from a dangerously abusive environment, as evidenced by the many scars on his skinny body. I lived at the time in a huge, largely empty loft space in a building filled with creative folk—a marvelous multicultural gang of actors, painters, dancers, lighting designers, and even a circus aerialist. And one stunned little boy. He was suddenly air-dropped from the violent streets and housing projects of Red Hook to a magical carnival in the Land of Oz. Everybody played with him, talked to him, tickled him, taught him all manner of cool things, and loved him, and the boy with the broken spirit grew roots and tender shoots and blossomed.

Some months after he came to live with me, Omar dreamt that the structural pillars in our loft and those on the floors above and below us were really one gigantic tree trunk that grew up through the seven-story building, all the way to the sky. He saw his new home as a protected nest in an embracing Family Tree, the sacred Tree of Life. The tree's roots ran deep into the earth and its branches touched the clouds, grounding him and connecting him to a loving community of supportive souls. Living there made him feel safe for the first time in his life. Our home was his dream of heaven.

Today we live in real "there but for the grace of all that is good, go I" times. Those of us who have homes are very lucky, especially if our homes are safe, warm, and loving. There are more than sixty-five million refugees on the planet today who have been forced to leave their homes to escape political vagaries, terrorism, devastating climate events, and famine. There are people sleeping in the streets of American cities and in suburban parking lots. Ten percent of New York City school kids are homeless. Entire Caribbean islands have been evacuated after hurricanes, to go where? And those numbers do not take into account the untold numbers of animals, domestic and wild, who have been driven from their homes, as well.

There is so much that we can do to help those unfortunate souls in gratitude for the blessings of our home.

- The simplest way of offering support without even leaving home is to write a check to a refugee, rescue, or homeless aid organization.

- We can open our homes to foster or adopt pets displaced by disasters and now in shelters. We can open our homes to foster orphaned children, as well.

- We can open our suburban or rural homes for a few weeks in summer to host an inner-city child's Fresh Air Camp vacation. Or we can offer a room for a year to a visiting foreign student.

- We can open our homes for local functions that foster good community relations.

- We can work in our communities to make them official sanctuaries for those who need shelter.

- We can volunteer with Habitat for Humanity and other such organizations. We can help elderly or disabled neighbors do home maintenance chores.

- We can sponsor an immigrant individual or family and help them to settle into new surroundings.

- We could make Blessing Boxes. There is a lovely trend growing in popularity among good-hearted folks, many of them children, across the United States to create Blessing Boxes as a way to reach out with support to those living in hard situations in these hard times. These so-called boxes are newly constructed or repurposed cabinets fitted with shelves and a door of some sort, and filled with food staples, household supplies, and hygiene necessities. These Blessing Boxes are then placed outside on front lawns, sidewalks, and other public places, usually sporting a sign that invites anyone to "Help yourself to anything you need." Constantly replenished, these free good-will dispensaries offer basic sustenance to those who are homeless, and also give critical additional support to the elderly, new immigrants, and working families who live precariously, always one meager paycheck away from being homeless.

Having a home is a true blessing. It is incumbent upon us to share our good fortune in whatever way we can. "To acknowledge privilege is the first step in making it available for wider use," wrote the poet Audre Lorde. "Each of us is blessed in some particular way, whether we recognize our blessings or not. And each of us somewhere in our lives must clear a space within that blessing where s/he can call upon whatever resources are available … in the name of something that must be done." And certainly there is no shortage of opportunities to offer aid. When we open our homes or our hearts, we expand both.

> Sharing grief is half the sorrow, but happiness
> when shared is doubled.
> —Haitian Proverb

Charity begins at home!

Every day is a journey, and the
journey itself is home

—Matsuo Basho

CHAPTER 8

Home Away from Home

Even if your home is a safe place of comfort and refuge that you can return to at any time, it can still be quite upsetting to be removed from it for long or even short periods. Since time immemorial when people left home for an adventure or for some necessity, whether away for work, at camp, or on the battlefields, it has been customary to bring with them pictures and amulets of various sorts that hold precious domestic feelings and memories to serve as a conceptual umbilical connection to home.

Homesickness is suffered widely across cultures and reflects the intense emotional attachment that we humans have to our own personal homes, our native cultures, and our loved ones. Homesickness is described in the Old Testament Book of Psalms (137:1): "By the rivers of Babylon, there we sat down, yea, we wept, when we remembered Zion." Homer's *Odyssey* opens with Athena trying to persuade Zeus to bring the homesick Odysseus back home, because he was "longing for his wife and his homecoming." Journals and letters of explorers, colonists, immigrants, pioneers, soldiers, prisoners, boarding school students, and summer campers confirm that no matter the reason for being separated from home, the common response is the same profound longing for the familiarity of home sweet home.

If, as the saying goes, "wherever you hang your hat is home" is true, it is important that every space where you spend time provide a friendly, secure, and uplifting environment in order for your soul to feel at home wherever you are and for however long you are there. So unless you are a turtle, an armadillo, a snail, or a mollusk and literally carry your home on your back, or you are a nomad, a Gypsy caravanner, or RVer and drive your home where you are going, you will want to carry some essence of home with you when you are away from it, so that you can tap into the feeling of domestic comfort and support while you are away. And you can do that digitally these days with apps that show you what is going on in your home when you are not there.

ON THE JOB

Most of us spend the greater, if not the best, portion of our day at work, where the environment is often the opposite of cozy and sometimes downright nasty. It is not always possible, nor is it appropriate, to burn smudge or drum and chant in order to cleanse the energy in a work setting, no matter how much it might be needed. But there are many other, less obvious ways to establish a calm and centering ambience, which is infinitely more conducive to productivity and cooperation, even within a professional, public, or chaotic setting. You can benefit from the purifying qualities of sage, cedar, juniper, frankincense, and myrrh without the smoke by using essential oils. A tiny drop just below your nostrils can convey the same healing, cleansing, soothing aroma as the actual plants. These herbs and many others are also available as sprays. They smell a lot better than commercial chemical air fresheners and serve to purify the atmosphere both physically and energetically. A rose of Jericho is a perfect energy purifier for a private or communal office. Just place this dormant plant in a pretty bowl filled with water. It will open and work to collect and absorb any unsavory energy in your environment. And no one will have any idea of what you are doing—though they may comment on your unusual plant!

Some people prefer to work in an anonymous environment, but most of us like to have some personal touches in our surroundings, be they sentimental, spiritual, or silly. These special images and objects are, like a fingerprint, stamps of identity. They are statements of ownership that ground us and remind us of who we really are, or aspire to be—not as we are defined by our job. You can, and probably already do, fill your cubicle or office with mementos of home, family, and friends, as well as travel memorabilia and an assortment of small items that amuse or inspire you—a special coffee cup, a nice pillow to sit on, a screen saver with a photo of your daughter's birthday party, a rock from your last hike. These treasures create a virtual home away from home, a spiritual safe haven in the midst of stressful surroundings. Your altars and amulets carry the energy of your home when you are at work or school and they keep you connected to a supportive homey energy whenever you need it during your day.

It is possible to create a lovely and effective altar even in a really small place—on the dashboard of your cab or truck, or on the inside of your locker door, for example. Schoolkids and workers alike decorate their lockers with pictures, magnets, inspirational quotes, and other personally relevant items. This practice offers instant cheer every time the door is opened. A desktop altar can be assembled with just one or two carefully chosen items—a candle, for example, to light with intention at the start of an assignment or project, as a mini meditation to clear your mind and help you focus on the task at hand.

You can create the same result by fashioning a small altar in a box, basket, or pouch that you can keep on a shelf or in a closet or drawer and access whenever you need to. Why not keep a collection of small natural items—stones, shells, acorns, pinecones, crystals, or dried flowers—hidden in a desk drawer to fondle when you are frazzled and longing to be outside in nature. This tiny ritual can function as a one-minute vacation to a favorite hideaway retreat.

There are ways to enlist your electronic devices as collaborators in your efforts to nourish your spirit while at work. You can easily adjust your screen saver with images of inspiration, a favorite quotation, an affirmation, a beautiful mandala, or a nature scene, and breathe it in when you turn your computer on. When you stop paying attention to it, change the image to keep your response fresh. You can also set an alarm (don't ask me how, I am a complete techno-poop) to remind you to take a break, take a walk, take a deep breath. I love this feature. It has trained me to get up and move around every hour. And even though it means interrupting my immediate attention on what I am doing, at the end of five minutes away from my work, my concentration is revitalized.

If you are a mail carrier, farmer, visiting nurse, or other occupation that keeps you on the move with no delineated workspace, you can carry special charms, amulets, and talismans in your purse, pocket, or briefcase to keep you connected to your personal life wherever you are. An amulet bag filled with small, meaningful items of spiritual significance is like an altar on the go. Just looking at or touching these sacred items puts you in mind of what is truly important to you. This gives you the same sense of inner peace, safety, and satisfaction that you feel in your own home. Most folks today, whatever their work environment, have created mobile altars on their cell phones filled with fond photos of family, friends, fun, favorite places, music, and objects, which they carry around with them, keeping a constant connection with what is meaningful. This device can serve as the essence of home in your pocket.

TAKING LEAVE

Your residence is your sanctuary, your refuge, your home base. It is the place where you prepare yourself to go out into the world and which then welcomes you when you return. Your home gives you energy. Or, if the atmosphere is stale, it saps your energy. In the same way, your energy, your spirit, has a palpable effect on your home. I know how vital it is for me to take some tangible reminders of home when I am away, which makes me wonder how my home feels when I am not there. (If a tree falls in the forest, does it make a sound if there is no one there to hear?) To ensure the continued reciprocal energy exchange with your house, take some reminders of home with you when you go and also leave some reminders of you at home. Prepare your place for your going. Try to leave it clean and orderly, which makes it so nice to return to. Bless your house with protection while you are gone. Bless the kitchen that feeds you, the bed that embraces you at night, your computer, your plants, your altars. Put out some fresh flowers to add fragrance and beauty to your home while you are away.

Our connection to home and family is a powerful protection that can sustain us when we are not there. As the dancer Bella Lewitsky said, "To move freely you must be deeply rooted." To be able to leave home, we have to believe that we can always return, that, yes, you *can* go home again. Even when leaving home to embark on a grand adventure, whether a vacation, a study year abroad, a new job, or a long-hoped-for emigration, parting can be "such sweet sorrow," bittersweet, and angst-ridden. In Hindu societies, family members tie a string around a traveler's wrist when s/he is embarking on a journey, so that they may retain their connection to the each other across time and space.

TRAVEL

In addition to the emotional turmoil of preparing, packing, and leaving for a journey, the process of traveling is fraught with insecurity, the unfamiliar, and potential impediments, all of which produce a certain amount of anxiety. The same can certainly be said about life itself. Travel, in fact, is an ancient and universal metaphor for life: life as path, as road, as voyage, as journey, as a trip.

Because of the uncertainty and potential perils of travel, people everywhere have always petitioned the Powers That Be for protection and smooth passage.

May calm be spread around you
May the sea glisten like greenstone
and the shimmer of summer
dance along your path.
—Maori

May the hills lie low
may the sloughs fill up, in thy way
May all evil sleep
may all good awake, in thy way.
—Scottish

In the house made of dawn
In the story made of dawn
On the trail of dawn....
It is finished in beauty in
the house of evening light
From the story made of evening light
On the trail of evening light.
—Navajo

Ten thousand things bright
ten thousand miles/ no dust,
water and sky one color
houses shining along your road.
—Chinese

May you have warm words on a cool evening,
a full moon on a dark night,
and a smooth road all the way to your door.
—Irish

BLESS THE ROAD

Whether traveling by foot, by animal, or by motorized vehicle, a smooth road is essential for a safe journey. When road travel becomes hazardous, a blessing is called for. When the N1 road in the Limpopo province of South Africa became the site of a radical increase in accident fatalities a while ago, a large group of traditional healers gathered to perform a cleansing ceremony to reduce the carnage. The president of the healers association explained, "We are healing this road of death, so that motorists will be safe. As things stand now, the N1 reeks of blood."

The towns of Wanneroo and Rockingham in Western Australia celebrate annual Blessings of the Roads to ensure safe driving and to honor the road workers and police who keep them safe.

The village of Baan Nong Kung in Thailand was founded in 1932, and as a gesture of gratitude and blessing, the residents erected a spirit house decorated with elephant and horse sculptures and planted it right in the middle of the main thoroughfare, which was a dirt road. Some seventy-five years later, the road was widened and paved and the spirit house stayed in the center. One motorist was so disgusted by having it in the way of efficient traffic flow that he loudly ridiculed the spirit house. On his way home he was killed by a ten-wheeler truck and became the first in a long line of traffic deaths. A road construction worker also offended the spirit house, immediately after which he was run over by a tractor. Many people died after that, so the headman ruled that since the spirit house has always kept us safe, mocking it will not be allowed, and since then no one else has died on that road.

Washing of the Road ceremonies are celebrated every year in early September in Brazil. The Lavagem is a mystic tradition that was most likely begun in the early nineteenth century in the Bahia province. The faithful still walk in an eight-kilometer procession to the Bonfim Church, where the slaves were once forced to scrub the path and steps that lead to it. Slavery was abolished in 1880, but the washing with floral water, the dancing and singing of Yoruban chants continue. This cleansing ritual has now hit the streets in Manhattan and in Newark, New Jersey. The Lavagem parade of 46th Street in Manhattan's Little Brazil is an exuberant celebration of both Brazilian independence from Portugal and slave emancipation. It is a purification rite that washes away the tears and sins of the past.

VEHICLES

Animals are the oldest form of transportation, after human feet. And the impulse to elicit blessings for a secure ride is just as old. Horses, donkeys, water buffalo, and elephants are commonly honored by being decorated and blessed. This Equine Blessing comes from the Palio, the famous horse race held annually in Siena, Italy, since 1310:

Bless these beasts of burden.
May our steeds be swift of foot, calm of nature,
Strong in body, and sound in mind.
Give them the gift of a smooth gait.
Bestow them with exceptional health and long life.
Honor us with their presence, and make us worthy stewards.

The Arabic word *dua* means "to call out," "to summon." An Islamic *dua* to petition for the protection of an animal and rider is: "If you buy a camel, then you should take hold of its hump and say a *dua*, 'O Allah, I ask You for the goodness within her and the goodness that you have made her inclined towards, and I seek refuge with You from the evil within her and the evil that you have made her inclined towards.'" This same *dua* is now used to bless new cars.

People around the world are careful to consecrate every mode of motorized transportation. Religious clergy and traditional spiritual practitioners are commonly asked to perform a ceremony that ensures safety and luck by praying, chanting, sprinkling holy water, fanning perfumed smoke, drawing signs and symbols on the vehicle, and adorning it with flowers. In Thailand, Buddhist priests regularly bless new cars, motorbikes, and even new Thai Airways jets. In the Philippines, it is thought to be especially lucky to have a Catholic priest bless your jeep, car, or motorcycle on Palm or Easter Sunday.

At Copacabana near Lake Titicaca, Bolivia, owners decorate their cars, taxis, and buses with flower garlands, wreaths, and confetti, then line up for a weekly ceremony called *La Bendición de Movilidades*, "The Blessing of the

Vehicles." After the Blessing ceremony, vehicle owners and their families celebrate with champagne and fireworks. In the United States, motorcycle blessings are quite popular and many states host huge gatherings of riders each year to bless the cycles, the riders, and their friends to keep them safe and accident-free. This decades-long practice has spawned a national network of bike blessings, including blessings for bicycles, the first of which was held in 1999 at St. John the Divine Cathedral in New York City.

A Car Puja is a multi-part Hindu ceremonial blessing of an automobile officiated by a *pujari* along with the owner of the car.

- Blessing hands are washed three times in holy water.

- Rice is sprinkled onto the front of the car.

- A swastika, the ancient symbol that means "to be well" (not to be confused with the backward-facing Nazi symbol) is drawn on the hood of the car with the third finger of the right hand, using turmeric powder mixed with water or sandalwood paste.

- More rice is sprinkled while repeating holy mantras, including eleven of the 1,008 names of Ganesha, the elephant-god remover of obstacles.

- Incense sticks are lit and then circled around the swastika symbol three times in a clockwise movement, and then circled around the steering wheel in the same manner, while mantras are recited.

- A small Ganesha idol is blessed with holy water and installed on the dashboard to the right of the steering wheel so that it is visible to the driver.

- A coconut is then broken near the right front wheel and the milk sprinkled on the tire.

- The last step involves placing a lemon on the ground just in front of each tire and then driving over them three times in a circle until they are squashed. The breaking lemons symbolize the ridding of bad influences from the vehicle.

Of course you will want to bless your own car for safety, dependability, and pleasure. While you are at it, personalize your car by hanging good luck charms from the rear view mirror or create a dashboard altar. It has recently become popular for Jews to attach auto mezuzahs to their cars. Throughout the Third World folks sport elaborate colorful altars on the dashboards of cars, trucks, and buses. These are typically decorated with holy images, fresh or plastic flowers, statuettes of saints held erect by magnets, and all manner of lucky charms.

The blessing of boats and fleets is an ancient tradition, and still a very important event in coastal communities. Folks who use boats to fish, to transport goods, and to travel are understandably inclined to bless their vessels for safety and good luck. Several years ago I was called upon by the Governor of New York to offer a Blessing of the Fleet on the quadricentennial celebration of Henry Hudson's voyage from Amsterdam to the New World, where he founded New Amsterdam, New York City. A huge flotilla was led by a replica of Hudson's ship, the *Half Moon*, followed by Pete Seeger's boat, *Clearwater*; the NYC Police and Fire boats; and a long parade of private yachts, sailboats, and row boats, canoes and kayaks. I sprayed each vessel with my collection of World Blessing Water.

The tradition of christening a new ship with spirits of the potable sort dates way back. The ancient Greeks wore olive-branch wreaths around their heads, drank wine to honor the gods, and poured water on the new boat to bless it. The Babylonians sacrificed an ox, the Turks sacrificed a sheep, and the Vikings and Tahitians offered up human blood. The USS *Constitution* was launched in 1797 by the Captain's breaking a bottle of Madeira wine on its bow. The USS *Hartford* was christened three times, with water from the Atlantic Ocean, the Connecticut River, and Hartford Spring. But since the christening of the USS *Maine* in 1890, champagne has been the holy water of choice.

> May the tide
> that is entering even now
> the lip of our understanding
> carry you out
> beyond the face of fear
> may you kiss
> the wind then turn from it
> certain that it will
> love you back
> may you
> open your eyes to water
> water waving forever
> and may you in
> your innocence
> sail through this to that

—Lucille Clifton, *Blessing the Boats*

When I leave for a trip of any distance, by any mode of transportation, I have a whole series of little protective rituals to help get me from point A to point B in one piece. Before I leave my house, I bless myself on the back of my neck, a point of great vulnerability. I also bless my home, my animals, and my altars to be safe in my absence. I bless my car and my dashboard altar, as well as my dog and any other passengers or drivers. If I am flying, I bless myself the minute I get to the airport with a swig of vodka that I carry with me in an antique flask. And upon entering the plane, I bless that, too, as I casually rub its body with protection oil as I enter.

Though I fly, I soar, I zoom through the skies in my dreams and in my shamanic journeys, I am not a great flyer on planes. So when I do venture onto an aircraft, I always carry my precious amulet bag with me. This is a pink silk brocade Chinese packet filled to capacity with the charms and totems that inspire, calm, and empower me wherever I may be. Just feeling its considerable bursting-at-the-seams weight in my purse gives me confidence and a sense of security.

A few years ago, while waiting anxiously for a flight, I reached for my pocketbook only to discover, to my absolute horror, that I did not have my amulet bag with me. Oh no! Panic! What to do? I was determined to reassemble my amulets and recreate my altar in my mind. That way, I might still connect with and concentrate on its power. So I removed myself to the cocktail lounge, where I sat at a table and summoned up the contents of my travel altar one by one, then listed them in my notebook:

- A little tin airplane with a black silk tassel. The one my five-year-old niece told me was going to help me fly.

- A crow's foot.

- A gold pin that says ritual.

- A piece of polished moose horn.

- A city stone.

- An Egyptian scarab.

- A lock of my dog's hair.

- A crown feather from my bird.

- An amethyst pyramid to focus my intuitive senses.

- My rainbow crystal to channel light.

- A citrine crystal to mediate dark.

- A peonía seed for power.

- A cowry shell for creation.

- A blue ball for purity.

- A worry doll to take away my fear.

- A copper-lidded jar filled with healing soil from Chimayó.

- Medals of Mother Goddesses.

- And so on.

Recalling each magical charm and sketching them on paper made me feel much better. There they were, all present and accounted for. I turned the list over and inscribed my affirmation on the other side:

I am safe.
I am calm.
I am centered.
I am at home in my heart.

I didn't have a candle, so I lit a bar match to ignite my intentions, and I toasted them with another sip of vodka. Then I folded my list into my pocket and went to board my plane. I stepped into the skyway that afternoon with the same sacred calm and sense of cosmic rightness that I always feel after praying at my altar. I was connected and protected. And I actually enjoyed my flight.

TEMPORARY ACCOMMODATIONS

*I long, as does every human being, to be at home
wherever I find myself.*
—Maya Angelou

Travel can be a great adventure, but it can also be discombobulating. Once you get where you are going, you need shelter and sustenance, for your emotions and spirit, as well as for your physical requirements. If you are backpacking, tent or van camping, or traveling in a motor home, you can create any kind of ambience you want, making the space your own desired domain. This is not quite as easy when staying in a hotel, motel, hostel, dormitory, bed-and-breakfast, train, or ship cabin. Even if you are staying for just one night, you will want to occupy the space and feel comfortable and centered while you are there.

The same concepts and practices for creating a sacred space in your home also apply to making temporary domiciles homey. The canned air in planes and many motels doesn't move, and neither does the energy, which gets stagnant and stultifying. If you are staying in a no smoking room you can't burn any herbs to clear the air, but, again, a rose of Jericho is the perfect travel energy purifier. This tennis ball–sized dry plant can be packed in a Ziploc bag in even the smallest carry-on case. Put it in water when you first get to your room and it will open up and absorb any bad energy from past guests. Then when you are preparing to leave, take it out of the water, stick it back in the bag, and it will be ready to use again when you need it next.

There is great benefit in intentionally choosing what surrounds you. This includes how the furniture is positioned. It amazes me that in many "rooms with a view" the bed is set perpendicular to the window, or backed against it, so that the view you paid extra for is obscured. However, the opposite is too true, as well. The bed always seems to face the window if it looks out onto the parking lot or a mall or the freeway! I can't count how many times I have spent the first half-hour in a hotel room rearranging the furniture. And it has been worth every second of effort to be able to relax in a room that feels right and offers something lovely to look at.

Simple gestures can create huge mood shifts. A picture of a dear one on the night table, an affirmation taped to the bathroom mirror, a crystal under your pillow, your journal, a favorite book, your own music playlist all elicit a sense of belonging and help you feel more connected to what's truly meaningful in your life while you are separated from it. You can transform an anonymous, generic, or downright ugly decor with a couple of easy-to-pack scarves, shawls, or pashminas. A favorite scarf draped over a lamp shade, a shawl in a pleasing color laid out on a hideous couch or chair, or hung over the television or an awful painting, puts your aesthetic stamp on the surroundings, making you feel much more like yourself. If you bring a few spiritual items from your altars at home, you can set out a small version on top of the desk, dresser, or bathroom counter where you will see it. When I am in residence at a retreat center for some amount of time, I create more ornate altars incorporating candles, the contents of my amulet bag, and my ceremonial jewelry plus any lucky stones or pine cones I might find while there. And, of course, I smudge everything when I am allowed.

Even one simple *hygge* addition can transform any room into a welcoming personal space. A living plant or some flowers make any space more homey, as do animals. Some hotels will lend you a bowl of goldfish or even a cat to keep in your room. When my fairy-goddess daughter first came to spend the summers with me, she was three years old. To celebrate the occasion and make her visit special, I bought her a cheerful set of floral sheets to sleep on. They were for her and only for her. No one else who stayed in my guestroom used those sheets. And when, occasionally over the decades, the room was given over to a visitor for a few days, she happily made her bed on the couch using her own personal linens. Wherever she spread those sheets was home to her.

> Wherever you stand, be the soul of that place.
> —Rumi

In biblical times, when the Jews were wandering in the wilderness after being expelled from Egypt, they built a portable sanctuary, or *mishkan*, that they could carry with them wherever they went. Having such a mobile sacred space while traveling is wonderful, and it becomes so much more essential when the room you are staying in is not for work or fun, but for some unpleasant necessity—a stay in a hospital, nursing home, or hospice, for instance. Studies show that when the elderly are moved, not of their own desire, into a nursing home and out of their own home, they are more vulnerable to death due to the stress of homesickness. The patient's dislike of the new nursing home seems to cancel out the better medical care that it can provide.

Even places such as these can be much more comforting, more supportive, and, ultimately, more healing by creating a nature-rich environment. Many long-term care establishments now have gardens to work or sit in for the huge pleasure of connecting with such a vibrant life force. Exposure to nature is healing for the spirit as well as the body. In 1984, a classic study found that patients recovered from surgery quicker if their hospital room looked out at a natural living environment compared to those who had no window or could only see a dead scene like a brick wall or a parking lot. Placing plants in hospital rooms also accelerates the rate of recovery, according to researchers at Kansas State University. Even posters depicting garden, forest, sky, or water scenes have a beneficial soothing effect.

> Nature is not a place to visit, it is home.
> —Gary Snyder

Institutional rooms can be made a great deal more pleasant if they reflect your aesthetic and spiritual sensibilities. Wearing your own pj's rather than a hospital gown, using a favorite perfume, covering the bed with a handmade afghan from home, having a display of pictures and altar items that speaks to who you are and what you hold sacred can mean a world of difference in an anonymous, sterile setting. Most care facilities encourage taping cards and pictures to the wall, and many have instituted programs of visiting dogs and cats to add a cheering experience. When I shattered my wrist while on vacation in Maine, the hospital allowed me to bring my dog into the emergency room, where she lay on my chest while I was being treated. And later, when I had surgery, I was able to bring my amulet bag into the operating room. If all hospitals had these humane practices, there would be much less need for anxiety and pain meds.

There are other rooms in other institutions that are even more traumatic and disorienting. Imagine the stress of being forced to live in a jail cell, a homeless shelter, a displaced persons or refugee camp, where you are separated not just from home but from every aspect of life as you knew it. Millions of people have been forced out of their homes by natural disasters or human violence with only the clothes they are wearing and whatever they happen to have in their pockets. In an emergency there is no time to take anything with you that you want or might need, and prisoners are not permitted most personal belongings. Harsh, crowded settings like these may offer shelter, but there is no privacy, no quiet, no control.

In circumstances like these, your sacred altar *mishkan* needs to be conceptual. Home is where you are welcomed, valued, and supported. When you are denied these emotional comforts, you must find your home within yourself—your inner home, the container that houses the entire cache of spiritual support skills that you have cultivated over time. The home you occupy in your deepest soul center, your internal *querencia*, your mobile *sitio*, your connection to spirit, your home in the universe is all you have to help you survive such a nightmare. In these sorts of situations, *you* are the sacred space! Wherever you go, whatever you do can be holy.

Heading towards that inner home will take you places—
both inside yourself and in the external world—
which your heart will recognize as its native environment,
even though you have never been there before.
—Martha Beck

Wherever you roam is home.

The words "blessing" and "blood" spring from
the same root in the English language.
This allows us to think of blessing as a life-giving
blood-stream, a current of spiritual energy
circulating through the universe.

—Brother David Steindl-Rast
99 Blessings: An Invitation to Life

CHAPTER 9

Homework

Probably the oldest substance used for blessings was blood, as it represents the animated pulsing life force. Blood from animal sacrifice is still used widely today in a variety of ceremonies practiced around the world. In many places, the flowing blood from trees, the sap and resin, are considered holy and used ceremonially. There are, in addition, a great many other common materials used in Blessing rituals that are gathered from the living plant kingdom: leaves, flowers, grasses, twigs, bark, and sticks, as well as minerals from the earth.

Here is a list of some of the more popular tools and supplies used around the world for spiritual cleansing and blessing.

BLESSING AGENTS

Water and/or smoke are the most common substances used to clear a space of negative energy and bless it for good. Together, they represent the four elements of nature.

Water is the source and essential sustenance of life. We live on a planet that is nearly three quarters water. Our bodies are composed of an average of one half to three quarters water, and we each spent approximately three quarters of a year immersed in womb waters. We even had gills at one point in our development long ago. We live on a blue water planet and we are aquatic beings. Water is a symbol of life and, as such, it is intrinsically holy. Blessing with water is universal. We bathe for physical cleanliness, but also for psychological and spiritual cleansing. The clergy of many traditions ceremonially cleanse individuals, animals, vehicles, homes, and places of worship by sprinkling holy water or waters infused with herbs or flowers along with their prayers. This sprinkling of blessings is called "spurging." I have a collection of what I call "World Water," a mixture of water from more than fifty holy sites and healing wells from all seven continents. I use this potent elixir for personal and public blessing ceremonies of all kinds.

We know that water has great powers of healing
and cleansing, and we also know that water is vulnerable
to contamination and pollution. Blessed be the water.
—Starhawk, *The Earth Path*

Smoke is the alchemical result of combining the other three elements: something of the earth—leaves, grasses, flowers, tree bark, roots, sticks, sap, or resin—is burned with fire, thus producing fragrant air, or "holy smoke!" Some peoples contain the fire in an abalone or other shell, which then symbolically adds water to the powerful mix, unifying all four elements. Spreading this healing smoke with a feather or a fan is called smudging. Chief Wise Owl Blue Feather explains, "The smoke attaches itself to negative energy and as it clears it takes the negative energy with it, releasing it into another space to be regenerated."

This method of purification has long been employed by the indigenous peoples of the Americas in a wide assortment of ceremonies to release unwanted energy and invite in the benevolent spirits. The smoke also facilitates a positive, reverent, and grateful spirit, as this popular Native American saying demonstrates: "Give thanks for unknown blessings already on their way."

AGENTS FOR CLEANSING AND PURIFICATION

Clean your room well, for good spirits
will not live where there is dirt.
—Shaker Saying

- Does the energy in your home feel heavy? Dark? Unsettling? Upsetting?

- Is there a specific object or room or corner that feels this way?

- Do you feel foggy, constricted, blocked?

- Is anyone in your household feeling or projecting negative vibes?

- What needs to come clean? In your house? In your psyche?

Camphor is a white crystalline substance, obtained from the Cinnamum camphora tree, which is native to south China, Taiwan, Japan, Korea, and Vietnam. Camphor has been used for many centuries as a component of purifying incense. It not only destroys harmful energy, it also repels insects and kills fleas. In India, *Kapur*, as it is known in Hindi, is burnt to purify the energies in a place and to freshen the air. The burning of camphor is symbolic of the destruction of human ego, because when it burns, it slowly disappears without leaving any residue, taking all negativity with it. Camphor can be burnt on a hot coal, dissolved in water, or used dry by placing some in the corners of the room or under sofa and chair cushions to cleanse the energy of anyone who sits there.

- Put a piece of camphor in a bowl of water, as you would a blue ball. Or . . .

- Burn a chunk on a hot coal. Or . . .

- Place dry camphor under sofa or chair cushions to collect left unwanted energy.

Cedar is a guardian plant that drives out negative energy and clears sacred space. The smoke is used to cleanse ritual tools and open the soul before calling upon the healing spirits. Cedar branches cover the floor of many sweat lodges, where ceremonies for the purification of body and spirit are held. The peoples of the Pacific Northwest swish branches of cedar through the air to cleanse an indoor space. These tribes consider cedar to be sacred, possessing ancient wisdom. When a cedar tree is old or dies, it is honored with offerings and prayers of gratitude.

A powerful repellant of energetic negativity, cedar is also commonly used in chests and closets to ward off destructive insects.

- Burn bundles of dried cedar by lighting one end. Or . . .

- Burn a small amount on a hot coal. Or . . .

- Use a cedar branch to sprinkle holy water in blessing.

Hyssop is a brightly colored flowering shrub native to southern Europe, the Middle East, and the area surrounding the Caspian Sea. It has been used as an energy cleanser since antiquity. Priests in ancient Egypt used it for spiritual purification. In the Old Testament Book of Leviticus, God commands people to use hyssop in the ceremonial cleansing of people and houses. In Renaissance Europe, the leaves and flowers were strewn around the house, particularly in sickrooms, as an air freshener that rids the place of disease-carrying spirits. Today hyssop is most often steeped in water and used to consecrate ritual tools and made into charms to clear negativity and evil spirits from a home.

- Soak the flowers in water to use in a purification ritual. Or . . .

- Burn the dried leaves in a heat-resistant bowl, shell, or cauldron.

Salt has been used for thousands of years to cleanse germs, to preserve foods, and also to purify tainted energy.

It is commonly spread across thresholds and sprinkled around the perimeter of rooms, homes, and properties to dispel unwanted psychic disturbances and delineate a safe space. Catholic holy water includes the addition of blessed salt, making the protective qualities of the water so much stronger. Native Hawaiians use unrefined mineral-rich sea Alaea salt for rituals of healing and in sacred ceremonies to purify, cleanse, and bless their tools and canoes. Used in a bath or carried in a pocket, pink Himalayan salt is an aura cleanser. When a candle is lit in a hollowed-out chunk, it heats the salt, which then emits negative ions that freshen the surrounding atmosphere, as well as the internal disposition. Black salt, known as sal negro, Witches Salt, Drive Away Salt, Voodoo Salt, and Santeria Salt, is used throughout the Caribbean Islands and much of South America. This is ordinary salt that has been doctored with additional protective elements. Scattered like any salt, black salt is used to banish the most hostile people and resistant harmful energies, hexes, and jinxes, and to keep them far away.

Basic Recipe for Black Salt

2 parts sea salt

1 part burnt carbon scrapings from a cast iron skillet or pot

1 part fine ash from your fireplace or altar

1 part finely ground black pepper

- Place some black salt outside the door or under the chair of someone you would like to leave your house—an overstayed guest or irritating roommate, for example.

Sandalwood, a semiparasitic tree growing on the roots of other trees, is found throughout Southeast Asia and the islands of the South Pacific. Both the wood and the roots produce a yellow aromatic oil that stays fragrant for many years. The wood is ceremonially burned to exorcise any negativity from the atmosphere. Sandalwood is held sacred to Hindus, who grind the wood into a paste, which is used to mark religious utensils, to decorate the icons of the deities, and to purify the mind during meditation and ceremonies. Zoroastrian priests offer sandalwood twigs to the urn in the fire temple, where the holy cleansing flames are kept constantly burning for the purification of all souls.

- Burn chips of sandalwood for the smoke. Or . . .

- Use sandalwood oil for the same results.

Sound is universally used to rout out and repel negative forces. The noise scares the bad spirits away. Cultures around the world bang drums, ring bells, blow horns, and set off fireworks at whatever New Year they celebrate to prevent stale and harmful energy from following them over the threshold into the fresh New Year. Rattles, maracas, shekeres, and tambourines not only keep the rhythm in spiritual ceremonies and church services, they serve to scare away the devil. These sound makers are like rattlesnake rattles, sending out a clear warning signal: "This is sacred space. Intruder energy beware!" Clapping hands, foot stamping, whistling, chanting, yodeling, and screaming all serve the same purpose.

• Have fun.

Thyme is native to the Mediterranean region, from which it was spread throughout Europe by the Roman armies. Thyme is a mighty fighter of negative energy and drives all vestiges away. The Roman soldiers added it to their bathwater to make them as strong, brave, and forceful as the plant. Burning thyme to cleanse a room brings a hearty energy of health and vitality to the house. Smudging with thyme vanquishes nightmares and dispels melancholy, hopelessness, depression, and other bothersome negative vibrations, especially after a trauma or family tragedy or during a long sickness. It repels insects, too.

• Dry the leaves and burn them on a hot coal.

White sage, as it is commonly known, is properly called "salvia," meaning, "to heal" from the Latin. White sage grows wild in the Great Plains across the north of the United States and the southern Canadian provinces. One of the four sacred herbs of the indigenous peoples of North America, white sage is used widely in smudging ceremonies to drive out dark forces and destructive influences in people and places. The smoke from burning the dry leaves facilitates a deep metaphysical cleansing and release from whatever might trouble the mind, such as worry, stress, hard feelings, and unhealthy attachments. The smoke releases large amounts of negative ions into the atmosphere, actually changing the chemical composition of the air. This atmospheric change is associated with a lighter and freer, more positive mood, according to scientific research, confirming what Native Americans have long known and practiced.

- Burn bundles of dried sage by lighting one end. Or . . .

- Burn a small amount on a hot coal.

May this person and space be washed clean by the smoke of these fragrant herbs. And may that same smoke carry our prayers spirally to the heavens.
—Native American Smudging Prayer

*Yerba santa, also known as Holy Weed, Mountain Balm, Gum Bush, Bear's Weed, Sacred Herb, and Sacred Weed, is a shrub that grows in the mountainous regions of the southwestern United States and northern Mexico. Yerba santa, meaning "sacred herb," is held to be holy by local native peoples, who traditionally carried some in their medicine bags to burn whenever purification was called for. Yerba santa smoke is used to cleanse impure, unhealthy energies that can create illness. It is effective in the release of emotional pain stored in the heart chakra. The uplifting scent reduces fear and emotional injuries, and aids in repairing inappropriate behavior, which often leads to disease. Burned in the sickroom, its pleasant aroma helps dispel hostile spirits that might have caused the illness.

- Burn bundles of dried yerba santa by lighting one end. Or . . .

- Burn a small amount on a hot coal.

AGENTS FOR PROTECTION

A blessing is a circle of light drawn around a person
to protect, heal, and strengthen.
—John O'Donohue, *Anam Cara*

- Do you feel safe in your home?

- What makes you feel insecure?

- What scares or worries you?

- Is there a particular spot that feels vulnerable?

- Bless that spot with protection.

Aloe vera is a succulent plant that grows wild in tropical climates around the world and is also cultivated for medicinal purposes. Just having a potted aloe plant in the home provides protection for all who live there. It is believed that hanging an aloe plant over or behind your door wards off evil influences. Aloe is especially effective in preventing domestic accidents and misfortunes, particularly burns. Folk legends describe the aloe as a sort of energetic bellwether, saying that if the plant flourishes, good things will come to the home, and if it withers, it signals a lot of negativity in the place. Ingesting aloe protects the immune system and thus wards off disease.

- Give it light and water.

Basil is possibly native to India, where it has been cultivated for more than five thousand years. Holy basil is held to be sacred in India, where many Hindu households keep their own basil plant, pray to it, and keep a lamp burning by it at night to ensure spiritual and physical safekeeping. Basil was used in English folk magic to ward off harmful spells as well as to keep away pests. In Haiti, Santeria practitioners fumigate with basil smoke to remove spirits from a home. In South America people keep a bit of basil in each room to protect the home and family. And when they leave the house, they rub some basil on their forehead for protection.

- Burn bundles of dried basil. Or . . .

- Burn a small amount on a hot coal. Or . . .

- Soak fresh leaves in water and spray it around what you want protected.

> Where Basil grows, no evil goes!
> Where Basil is, no evil lives.
> —Folk Saying

Blue Balls, or *Anil Modamo*, is widely used in protection rituals in many areas of the world. This is laundry bluing, the same substance that our mothers and grandmothers bought in bottles or little wrapped cubes to add to their wash for purity. There is a very fine line between purification and protection. If the atmosphere and energy is clean, there can be no place for negative spirit to hide. Today Anil is available as little Blue Balls, which are dipped in water to create a sort of paint that is used to draw protective boundaries around doors and windows, emphatic lines of protection past which unwanted energy cannot pass.

A bowl of water with a Blue Ball in it absorbs any residual or accumulating negativity in the room. Flush the sullied water away periodically, then add fresh water and a new Blue Ball to maintain a well-protected space.

- Float a ball. Or . . .

- Use it as nonpermanent paint to draw symbols.

Juniper is an evergreen shrub found on mountains and heaths throughout Europe, Southwest Asia, and North America. A powerful protector when planted by the entrance or hung at the door, juniper will guard a home and the occupants against evil forces, evil people, ghosts, and thieves. Pinning a sprig of juniper on clothing is believed to protect the wearer from accidents, snakes, and wild animal attacks. Dried juniper berries can be strung together like beads and then worn as protective amulets. In Scotland, houses are thoroughly scoured at New Year, after which a burning branch of juniper is carried from room to room as a blessing for protection in the coming year.

- Burn bundles of dried juniper by lighting one end. Or . . .

- Burn a small amount on a hot coal. Or . . .

- Carry juniper seeds for protection.

Plants are widely used for home protection, both literally and symbolically. Holly, cactus, and other prickly plants are planted near the entrance of a house to protect and safeguard all who dwell there. Wreaths made of cinnamon, garlic, rosemary, and rowan are thought to keep a house safe from invasive spirits. Certain house plants work to protect the interior air quality: spider plants, snake plants, bamboo palm, flowering mums, peace lily, mother-in-laws-tongue, areca palm, reed palm, dwarf date palm, Boston fern, English ivy, Australian sword fern, rubber plant, weeping fig, pot mums, and Gerbera daisies are just a few.

Rose of Jericho is desert tumbleweed also known as the Resurrection Plant, because it is able to come back to life after years of dormancy. When placed in a small bowl of water, it opens to reveal a lovely vibrant green plant, which smells clean and fresh, like the forest after a rain. And, like rain, it emits negative ions, which cleanse the air. A rose of Jericho in a bowl of water will, like the Blue Balls, continue to protect a space by continually absorbing any unwanted energy, like a sin eater. When the water evaporates, the rose closes again, swallowing and digesting unwanted energy. I think of this amazing perpetual plant as a spiritual Venus flytrap. When it returns to being a dried-up ball, its dormant state, replenish the water and it will open up again. Folk wisdom tells us that "a house where the rose of Jericho is kept will be a blessed house!"

- Place your rose of Jericho in a bowl slightly bigger than it is. Fill the bowl with water. The rose will open. It will absorb all negativity from your environment. When the water evaporates, the rose will dry out and close, digesting/disposing of all the negative energy that it has collected. When the rose is completely dry, add more water. This is important, since the rose is a desert plant and too much water can cause it to grow mold.

Vetiver is a perennial grasslike plant indigenous to the Himalayan mountains, southern India, Sri Lanka, and Malaysia, where Gods and idols are honored with garlands made of vetiver grass. The thin aromatic roots are burned as incense. The fragrant aroma gives protection against negativity of all kinds, including anger, grief, stress, bad dreams, and age-old traumas stored in the subconscious. Vetiver has been woven into screens, mats, and fans for thousands of years to repel insects, rats, thieves, and the intense tropical sun, as well as malevolent psychic invasion.

- Burn the roots on a hot coal.

AGENTS FOR SPIRITUAL ELEVATION

Spirituality is meant to take us beyond our tribal identity into a domain of awareness that is more universal.
—Deepak Chopra

Copal is a saplike plant resin that has been burned for thousands of years in smudging ceremonies by the indigenous cultures of Central and South America. Copal is used traditionally as a sacred offering to the Great Spirits with blessings of gratitude. Copal was burned in great quantities atop the Aztec and Mayan pyramids and in ancient Mexican burial grounds. The aroma of smoking copal opens the heart space and expands consciousness, creating a pathway that allows humans to unite with the greater universe and everything in it. The lovely white smoke is a connecting thread between the worlds, between heaven and earth and between humans, the deities, and the natural forces, thus facilitating intuitive and psychic communication.

- Burn a chunk of copal on a hot coal.

Frankincense is probably the oldest and most widely used incense in the world. It dates back to Egypt and Babylonia and spread to Africa, Israel, Greece, Rome, Japan, China, and India, where both Hindus and Buddhists still burn it in their rituals and festivals. The aromatic smoke clears the energy field and lifts the spirit to a higher level, which is why it is still widely burned in the Catholic Church. It strengthens one's spiritual connection and centeredness, so it is a great aid for meditation, visualization, and creativity. Frankincense is used for creating a calm atmosphere that relaxes panic and relieves stress, tension, and hysteria, making healing possible on many levels. Science affirms that frankincense has a potent, positive effect on the brain.

- Burn a chunk of frankincense on a hot coal.

Jasmine, which means "Gift of God" in Persian, is native to tropical and temperate regions of Eurasia, Australasia, and Oceania. The delicate fragrance of the flowers is powerful in its ability to evoke calm, inner peace, divine beauty, and a compelling aura of love. Considered to be sacred, jasmine symbolizes innocence and purity of mind, which in turn promotes intuitive insight, creativity, and new ideas. In India, garlands woven with jasmine flowers adorn the temples and holy effigies and are offered to the deities. The Gods themselves are thought to be present within the flowers when they are used in ceremonies.

- Best used as is; place some fresh flowers in a vase. Or . . .

- As adornment of your altar. Or . . .

- Pin some in your hair.

Lavender is a small flowering shrub found across Europe, North Africa, South Asia, and the Cape Verde and Canary Islands. The smoke created by burning dried lavender flowers restores inner balance and creates a peaceful, tranquil, harmonious atmosphere, making it an excellent aid for meditation. Lavender, which means "to wash," does, indeed wash away any mental resistance, making it safe for the mind to open and feel free to soar to higher realms. The peaceful energy of lavender heightens psychic awareness and promotes dreaming, divination, and clairvoyance, and also enhances memory.

- Burn the dried flowers on a hot coal. Or . . .

- Place some under your pillow for a peaceful sleep. Or . . .

- Put some in your hot bath to relieve stress.

Mint is a hardy perennial growing across Europe, Africa, Asia, Australia, and North America. Though it smells great when fresh, the smell of burning mint is not agreeable. It is usually steeped in water, either to drink or to sprinkle as a blessing. Simply smelling the fresh aroma of mint calms the nerves and uplifts the spirit. Mint is invigorating and restorative, calling us to attention. It stills excess emotions; chases away depression, inertia, and laziness; opens the heart chakra; clears karmic issues; revives the mind; and renews a sense of hope. In all these ways, mint is very beneficial for soothing grief and was used in funerary rites in ancient Greece. The aroma of mint in the home is inviting to people, deities, the ancestors, and all helping spirits alike.

- Keep a live plant in the kitchen to keep the air fresh and invigorating.

Myrrh is a resin harvested from small thorny trees that grow in Saudi Arabia, Oman, Yemen, Somalia, Eritrea, and Ethiopia. The smoke has a spicy, earthy aroma that brings the astral realms closer to the earth, opening a passageway to spiritual awareness and enlightenment. Often burned in combination with frankincense, it enhances meditation and divination, restores clarity, and elevates the internal and environmental energies. Best of all, myrrh heals old wounds to the heart, so that it can remain open, yet protected, in order to welcome and receive love. Smudging with myrrh consecrates, purifies, and blesses sacred objects such as amulets, talismans, charms, icons, and magical tools.

- Burn on a hot coal.

Palo santo comes from a tree native to coastal South America. Its name means "holy wood," which indeed it is. For untold generations, the Incas and the shamans of the tribes throughout the Andes have burned it as a smudge to inspire spiritual purity and heightened consciousness. Its enticing aroma works to raise the vibrations of the body, as well as the atmosphere, and at the same time to keep the energy grounded. Its uplifting citrusy scent helps to evoke a deeper connection to the Earth and the divine source. This sacred wood is never cut from living trees, but is gathered from fallen dead branches that have lain on Mother Earth for four years.

- Just light the end of a stick to release the smoke.

Sweetgrass grows wild in the prairies and fields in the cooler northern regions of the United States and the southern provinces of Canada. It is considered to be the sacred hair of Mother Earth by the Native Peoples. The tall grass is harvested and then ceremonially braided into three strands, representing mind, body, and spirit, and also love, kindness, and honesty. When burned, the sweet musty smoke brings in the sweet gentle spirits of the universe. Its calming, relaxing effect feels like being swaddled in the protective mothering embrace of the goodness of being. When used to smudge people, the smoke is directed to clear the eyes, ears, heart, and body. Like a sacred medicine, it clears the vision, the awareness, the speech, and the action.

- You can light the end of the braid, but . . .

- It is safer and more economical to trim a short length and burn that on a hot coal.

This smoke from the sweetgrass will rise up to you,
and will spread throughout the universe.
Its fragrance will be known by the wingeds,
the four-leggeds and the two-leggeds,
for we understand that we are all relatives;
may all our brothers be tame and not fear us!
—High Hollow Horn

Tobacco is one of the four sacred plants, along with sage, cedar, and sweetgrass, used ceremonially by Native

Americans of many cultures to establish a relationship with the energies of the universe. It is believed that tobacco opens the door to the Creator and enables communication with the spirit world. Tradition says that this is so, since the plant's roots dig deeply into the earth, and its smoke rises high into the sky. When the Sacred Tobacco is burned in a pipe, the smoke is not inhaled, but released into the air. The dried leaves are also offered by sprinkling them directly on the ground, on the water, on the mother drum, scattering on the winds at dawn, gifting to honored teachers, healers, elders, and ancestors with gratitude for the gifts of life received.

- Burn a pinch on a hot coal. Or . . .

- Scatter some crumbled dried leaves on the ground to spread your blessing. Or . . .

- Place some in an amulet bag or medicine bundle to keep on your altar. Or . . .

- Offer some at a holy site.

- Do you feel a connection with All That Is?

- What do you aspire to?

- What are you grateful for?

- What is holy to you?

AGENTS FOR LUCK AND GOOD FORTUNE

Good night, and good luck.
—Edward R. Murrow

- Do you believe in luck?

- What represents good luck to you?

- Do you use lucky charms?

- What are they?

- What sort of luck do you need?

- How can you invite luck into your home?

Bamboo is a tropical grass that grows on every continent except Europe and Antarctica. Because it is an extremely fast-growing plant, it symbolizes growth and abundance; and because it proliferates far and wide, it is thought to stimulate growth and prosperity. In Asia, bamboo is brought into a new house to bless it with good fortune. Bamboo is the Chinese symbol of uprightness and an Indian symbol of friendship. The presence of bamboo in a home brightens the energy of the space, creating a palpable burst of strength and inspiration for the people living there. The aura of bamboo increases mental flexibility, spiritual growth, artistic talents, good health, luck, love, longevity, and happy family relations.

- Nurture it with water and light and watch it grow.

Bay, also known as Laurel, is an aromatic evergreen shrub native to Asia Minor and areas around the Mediterranean. This herb enhances psychic abilities. It is said that the Oracle at Delphi wore a crown of laurel, chewed the leaves, and inhaled bay smoke so that she would be open to receiving the visions sent to her by Apollo, the God of Prophecy. People today put bay leaves under their pillow to attract foresightful dreams and clairvoyance. It is traditional to write a wish or intention on a bay leaf and then burn it to make your heart's desire come true. In addition to divination, this herb brings great good fortune and success. The winners of the ancient Olympic games were once honored with wreaths woven with laurel leaves, whereas today's victors receive crowns fashioned from olive leaves.

> A house is made of walls and beams;
> a home is built with love and dreams.
> —William Arthur Ward
> *Thoughts of a Christian Optimist*

This is your home.
Cleanse it.
Protect it.
Love it.
Bless it.
And in return,
your home will
continue to bless you.

If there is righteousness in the heart,
there will be beauty in the character.
If there is beauty in the character,
there will be harmony in the house.
If there is harmony in the home,
there will be order in the nation.
When there is order in the nation,
there will be peace in the world.

—Confucius

APPENDIX

The blessing agents listed on pages 210 to 231 are available from www.MamaDonnasSpiritShop.com, as well as from a wide range of herbal emporiums, botanicas, and spiritual supply shops in your area and online.

Mama Donna also creates DIY House Blessing kits in a box filled with everything you need to cleanse and bless your home or office. Available at www.MamaDonnasSpiritShop.com.

A percentage of each sale of this book, as well as purchases of blessing agents from www.MamaDonnasSpiritShop.com, is donated to Habitat for Humanity.

ABOUT THE AUTHOR

Donna Henes is an internationally renowned urban shaman, contemporary ceremonialist, spiritual teacher, author, syndicated columnist, popular speaker, and workshop leader. She has published four previous books, a CD, and an acclaimed Ezine and writes for The Huffington Post, Beliefnet, and UPI Religion and Spirituality Forum. A noted ritual expert, she serves as a spirituality consultant for the television and film industry. Mama Donna, as she is affectionately called, maintains a ceremonial center, spirit shop, ritual practice, and consultancy in exotic Brooklyn, New York, where she offers intuitive tarot readings and spiritual counseling and works with individuals, groups, institutions, municipalities, and corporations to create meaningful ceremonies for every imaginable occasion.